I0454754

Live To be

100

with a sound Mind And Body

Dr. Rudy Kachmann

Copyright 2012 by Dr. Rudy Kachmann
All rights reserved.
ISBN: 1475216092
ISBN 13: 9781475216097

Contents

Longevity

WE SEEM TO THINK ABOUT how long we will or could live only when we buy life insurance or are getting into our senior years.

The trouble is that the building blocks of longevity are laid down when we are young; the foundations are even formed when we are in our mother's womb. What illnesses she has and what she eats have a tremendous effect on the size of our brain. Is she diabetic? Does she have other serious diseases that could affect us? Even when we're children, what we eat will have tremendous effect on our longevity.

Our genes are not the biggest determining factor of our longevity unless we trigger them with bad dietary and toxic habits. The "thrifty gene" that we acquired during our evolutionary history, especially Africans, South Americans, Micronesians, and Japanese, are a setup for bad eating habits and result in Western diseases. These thrifty genes trigger obesity, type II diabetes, vascular disease, cancer, and dementia in a great deal of our American population.

My plan is for you to have a goal of living to be one hundred, physically and mentally strong.

There are numerous societies and cultures where people live to be a hundred at two to ten times the rate we do. What they do is in my Longevity Mind-Body Index. I discuss the twenty-five recommendations in detail in separate chapters.

Scientists studied some of the areas in the world where people are more likely to be centenarians, and they wrote a book called *The Blue Zones.* I recommend you read that book and look at their website, bluezones.com. They also offer a test of thirty questions to estimate your longevity, and they give their recommendations on how to increase it.

You may have all the good habits already, but then again, many of us do not and need to increase the odds.

In many cultures, such as China, Japan, etc., medical care is concentrated on prevention and not on procedures as in our culture. My wellness center is inside a large, five-hundred-bed hospital, like a breath of fresh air. Many physicians walk by it every day but have never stopped in to see what we offer for their patients to get well without injections, medications, or operative procedures. We have cured many of their diabetes patients by teaching them a proper way of eating and exercising. Unfortunately the majority of Western medicine treats the disease after you have it instead of preventing you from getting it. Some might say people don't wish to change. I don't agree.

Seventy-five percent of people who see a doctor need only a "coach,"not a prescription, injection, or operation.

Scientific studies of twins indicate 75 percent of longevity is determined by our lifestyle and not by our genetic structure.

The fountain of youth has not been found. Ponce de Leon was looking for it in Florida in the 1500s, and people have been looking for it forever.

My Longevity Mind-Body Index puts you on a direct course to a happy, long life, the best you can do that nature will allow at this time.

The longest life recorded is 120, but this may change with bio- and nanotechnology, with advanced scientific and research going on all the time.

In 2002, fifty scientists made a huge statement that may not be true today: "There are no lifestyle changes, surgical procedures, vitamins, antioxidants, hormones, or techniques of genetic engineering available today that have been demonstrated to influence the process of aging."

The brutal reality about aging is that it has only an accelerator pedal. We have yet to discover whether a brake exists for people. The name of the game is to keep from pushing the accelerator pedal so hard that we speed up the aging process. The average American, however, by living a fast and furious lifestyle, pushes it too hard and too much.

It is my opinion that we can extend life ten to twenty years by following the principles of the Longevity Mind-Body Index and could save ourselves from sudden death by following the basic principles early in life.

Because of bio- and nanotechnology, our aging process and length of life expectancy may change. It has not changed much in thousands of years, but we are indeed getting at the micro level of biology. Then again, in fifty years of research on Alzheimer's disease, we have essentially made zero progress in terms of treatment and prevention. But things probably will change, and you may be around to see it happen in your lifetime.

Some scientists think immortality is within our grasp. Let's at least be open-minded about it. At least follow the twenty-five principles that will help us get the max out of life at this time. Do we have the knowledge and tools today to live forever? Clearly the answer is no. But when we looked at the rate of biotechnological change, essentially doubling every ten years, we have to say yes to improvement. Whether it will be dramatic or not remains to be seen.

If you let your body fall apart, you certainly won't live a long time, but if you constantly build on it and repair it quickly, you may achieve the max possible today. We are beginning to understand that aging is the single progression of a group of related biological processes. Strategies for reversing these aging processes using different combinations of biotechnology are starting to emerge. Some believe we will have means to stop and even reverse aging within the next two decades.

Some experts believe that within a decade we will be adding more than a year to life expectancy every year. Others still don't believe that at all. It'll be tough to improve on Mother Nature, especially in areas as basic as your own DNA. Then again we just discovered the DNA helix in 1954, and a lot has happened since that time. The rate of change is itself accelerating. As we look into the twenty-first century, nanotechnology will enable us to rebuild and expand our bodies and brains virtually any way we want from the information, resulting in remarkable gains, even in health. We certainly will find it worthwhile to remain healthy and vital today to experience this potentially remarkable century ahead.

The leading causes of death are heart disease, cancer, stroke, respiratory illnesses, kidney disease, liver disease, diabetes, and cancer. They did not appear out of the blue. They are the end result of processes that are decades in the making, based on what we eat and the lives we lead. Some societies have very little of these diseases because they eat different food.

The enemy may be us. It actually is us

Aging starts at birth. When your mother looks you in the eye, the process begins. It occurs in all species, including ours. We probably peak in our twenties and start to decline in our mid-forties. We start losing muscle mass and brain cells, and our pancreas secretes less insulin, etc.

No clear biological explanation of aging has been formed except the indices of disease. Some people say that aging is a loss of mental and physical abilities and that you are not designed to keep physical integrity forever.

Another theory involves your DNA and RNA, including your mitochondria. You start losing some of your DNA and RNA strands, called telomeres, as years go by, and that is an endpoint.

Other scientific evidence points to oxidative stress and electron damage. Overeating causes a lot of oxidative stress. All eating involves oxygen and metabolism. So you can see the affects obesity can have on your longevity.

At birth, your chance of living to be one hundred is about 1 percent. Certainly the chances increase as you get older, centenarians are the fastest-growing age group—much higher in some societies than others, depending on their habits. The older you are, the healthier you have been. I recently read a great book, *Fantastic Voyage* by Ray Kurzweil and Terry Grossman. They said scientists are developing "blood cell-sized submarines" called nano bots, whose key features are measured in nanometers, or billions of cells a meter, to be sent into the human body on vital health missions. Research like this actually is going on today, so you can see that progress indeed may occur in the future—but you can never be sure.

GENESIS 6:3
Then the Lord said, "My Spirit shall not abide in man forever, for he is flesh: his days shall be 120 years."

Longevity Mind-Body Index

HOW CAN YOU LIVE TO be a hundred and be of sound mind? It's a pretty good challenge, but attainable. I've gathered twenty-five strong recommendations and certainly could add a lot more, but they are the core recommendations based on my observations, reading, and research. I've gathered them in my Longevity Mind-Body Index (LMBI), and I have other recommendations at my Mind-Body Institute website.

What you eat is certainly the most important item on the list, throughout your life from the day you are born. If your mother breast-fed you, she gave you omega-3 and other supplements, all needed for the development of the best brain you can get. As Senator Tom Harkin said recently at a Senate hearing on education that education begins before conception. I thought it was a profound statement, based on a four-year study carried out under President Ronald Reagan's administration. *The Secret of the Nondiet* for adults is a book I wrote about a way of eating, not dieting. It results in excellent health, avoiding most of the well-known illnesses and diseases and builds a good brain for the future. I describe it in detail, with choices of vegetarian, vegan, flexitarian, and a high-density nutritarian way of eating. Flexitarian is an about 80 percent vegetarian or vegan way of eating.

Avoid injuries. Head injuries from concussions, contusions, blood clots, and especially repeated injuries can lead to neurologic complications, memory loss, and a shorter life span.

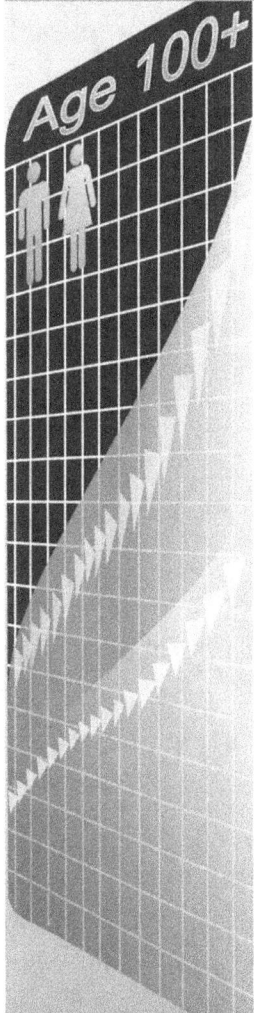

LONGEVITY MIND BODY INDEX

Age 100+

- Proper Eating
- Metabolic Panel–Once A Year
  - Complete blood count (cbc)
  - Lipid Profile
  - Glucose
  - PSA
  - TSH
  - Homocysteine
  - HB A1C
  - Vitamin D
  - Bone density test
  - CRP
- Exercise
- Normal BMI
- No Toxic Habits-(Smoking, Alcohol, Drug Use)
- Stress Reduction
- Avoid Risky Behaviors- (avoid falls and accidents)
- Normal Blood Pressure
- Purpose In Life
- Education- College and Adult
- Mindfulness
- Don't Retire- keep on working
- Positive Thinking
- Spirituality
- Memory-Protect and Improve (Computer Games)
  - *Visit Dr. Rudy's Brain Gym*
  - *www.kachmannmindbody.com (Brain Gym)*
- Hobbies
- Reading- 1 book per week
- Music-learn to play an instrument & go dancing
- Socialization-Make new friends
- DNA-Genes- avoid effect of thrifty genes
- Avoid obesity and diabetes
- Meditation-Yoga
- Proper Sleep Habits

As a neurosurgeon for forty years, I've treated many patients who suffered serious head injuries. As you would expect, this includes injuries from bicycles, motorcycles, three-wheelers, four-wheelers, airplanes, and boats, with results ranging from paralysis to death. The majority of these injuries could have been prevented if the people had been more thoughtful. Three-wheelers and four-wheelers are especially dangerous. Certainly, many of the bicycle and motorcycle accidents are not the fault of the people using them. Then again, they chose to use them, many times without helmets, and they are in constant danger to begin with because of trees and cars around them.

Just last night I saw what was probably a fatal motorcycle accident. The victim wore no helmet, his brain was running out of his ears, and he probably will be dead within a few days. Maybe his brain is dead already. Very sad; I see it all the time. The patient will no longer suffer, but his family will suffer forever. We have a good forty thousand motor vehicle deaths per year and thirty-seven thousand gun deaths per year. They certainly are not going to make it to a hundred. So avoiding accidents becomes important.

Repeated concussions starting at a young age can lead to dementia later in life. Amyloid bodies and neurofibrillary tangles typical of dementia develop even after mild concussions and contusions. Once we exceed our brain reserve, memory loss starts. Many football injuries—yes, even soccer injuries—have been studied, and there has been an increase in dementia years later. It has been proven. There have been a number of people in my community who've died from bicycle accidents. That's why we are raising a lot of money to build a bicycle path throughout the city. The families of the people who died are leading the effort, and many of us are helping financially.

I've been in neurosurgery forty-one years. I call motorcycles murder cycles. Recently a man and wife were riding on a motorcycle together, certainly a loving thing. They were hit by a car, and she is now lying in intensive care. She probably will live in a nursing home the rest of her life. Her husband came to my office, on his motorcycle, to talk about her. I noticed he rarely visits her. What can you say? The motorcycle riders overturned the helmet law in the state of Indiana; now they have freedom—freedom to die or live in the nursing home. Unfortunately, I see it all the time. I realize the helmet is not the only thing. It's the SUV and the 20 percent driving around with medication in them or texting down the road. Many times people don't see the bike or motorcycle because of inattention, and they are small vehicles to begin with.

I was almost run over by a teenager the other day while coming out of McDonald's after a cup of coffee. She was racing through the parking a lot, texting and not looking where she was going.

We lost about fifteen thousand people last year from self-inflicted gun injuries, suicides, accidents, and crime. That certainly will keep people from living to be a hundred also.

The rate of brain injuries increases sharply after age sixty because our senses are not as sharp. We don't see and hear as well as we once did, and we're becoming more imbalanced and take falls. Now many people are using aspirin, Plavix, or Coumadin for diseases they have accumulated over the years. These medications are very dangerous because if you fall, it becomes a major deal. Many times these falls lead to paralysis, living in a nursing home, or death. I see it almost daily; anticoagulants are a real problem. Plavix is particularly dangerous. If you're on it, double check to be sure you need it. I see many patients who should not be on it.

More than five million people will have head injuries this year, and nearly all could have been prevented. Protect your brain and watch what you're doing, especially if you are on blood thinners. Working on ladders or roofs is very dangerous. Riding on motorcycles and bicycles without helmets makes no sense, especially for young children. Use seatbelts at all times, and even if you've had just one drink, don't drive.

People who've blacked out for an hour or more after falling and had a head injury have a twofold increased risk for dementia. If they have the Apoe gene, it goes up tenfold.

Boxers and soccer players have an increased risk of dementia from repeated concussions. Unfortunately, a study on soccer players indicates they have a 30 percent increase rate of memory problems compared to normal people.

Studies done at UCLA by Dr. Bergsneider with PET scans found brain effects even in mild concussions. Dr. Houda noted that although a person may be able to walk, talk, and appear normal after a concussion, the brain may not be functioning normally. Can you imagine what could happen to a quarterback from repeated injuries?

People with increased brain reserves may demonstrate less effect for a period of time. Multiple small injuries have a cumulative effect and whittle away brain reserves. After a certain number of injuries, evidence of brain damage sets in. After head injuries, the brain immediately responds by forming amyloid plaques and neurofibrillary tangles as early as ten years of age.

In summary, avoiding injuries to that precious, three-pound brain is extremely important in avoiding memory loss and severe dementia in the future.

PROVERBS 3:16
Long life is in her right hand; in her left hand are riches and honor.

A Sense of Purpose

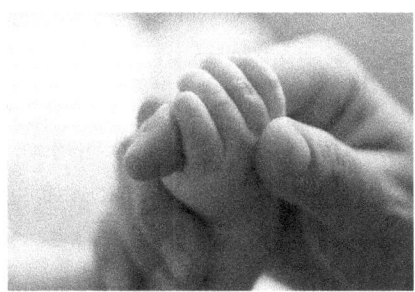

HOW CAN WE CONTINUE DOING THE SAME THING AND EXPECT A DIFFERENT OUTCOME?

WE ALL WANT A BETTER life, better health, financial gains, and a whole host of other things that we anticipate will give us that sense of purpose we so desire. How can we accomplish these huge goals? What will get us progressing in the right direction? As a wellness doctor and lecturer, I give both patient and the audience the education and the scientific background to stimulate change by teaching the wellness aspect of illness and disease. But is that really enough to get the job done? How motivating am I? Do my words lead to short-term or long-term changes in my listeners? I've certainly seen changes in my patients; some short-term and others long-term, and yet I suspect some others do not change at all. I practice what I preach, and I presume that to be motivating. And so I aim for long-term changes in my patients. Correlation is used to urge interaction, but it may be short-term. What you need is change that endures. You must be proactive if you plan to change your life. You need to start making changes immediately, or the commitment will leave you. Consistency in what you are doing can leave quickly as feelings interfere. Now you have another failed attempt, and you feel discouraged. A shaky commitment can get in the way of purposeful motivation. Creating a sense of purpose for your life and doing something to duplicate that is more likely to result in a permanent change, and you can accomplish your goal.

When you set out to create and accomplish, stimulated by this sense of purpose, you are most likely to cause these long-term changes within yourself. Motivation solves short-term problems, but for long-term results, you must find the root of your sense of purpose and renovate it. When we are fearful, we go for quick fixes. Drugs, cigarettes, and food are all chemicals that affect the mind for a quick fix. And of course, that only leads to more problems—poor health, family conflict, job loss...the list goes on and on. If you develop a sense of purpose in life, you are more likely to reach your long-term goal, and your subconscious mind will help you to get there. The famous cancer psychotherapist Dr. Lawrence LeShan found during forty-five years of treating cancer patients that if he could find or discover a purpose in life for his patient, he could double his or her lifespan and increase the likelihood of a spontaneous cure. A sense of purpose stimulates activity in the immune system, improving both longevity and cure rate.

Now sit down with a pencil and paper and write down what you are trying to accomplish, whether it be weight loss, transforming your appearance, improving family relations, making a career change, or getting rid of bad habits such as smoking and/or drinking. If you establish a sense of purpose to improve yourself, it is much more likely you will reach your goal and make it happen.

For example, although I am in my early seventies, I have created a sense of purpose by planning to be the national eighty-and-over tennis champ. I am already training for it. I take a tennis lesson once a week from the best player in town, do yoga and weight training three days a week, and play tennis at night on a regular basis. It has given me a reason to get out of bed, and I have a sense of great purpose. This is what motivates me. Additionally, I am writing books, creating DVDs, giving a great number of lectures on wellness, and practicing neurosurgery full-time. At seventy-three, I have developed a sense of purpose that is very motivating. I wake at 5:00 a.m. and start my day reading, writing, working out, and practicing my saxophone. By nine o'clock, I take a pause at Starbucks to meet friends and get ready for the day's work. I can't say it enough: I feel a great sense of purpose in helping others get well.

I hope you can find your purpose in life. It will motivate you to get the job done. Look for a sense of purpose, like getting in shape. For example, type 2 diabetes is curable in thirty days by eating the right foods. Or improve the relationships within your family. If you have self-induced physical problems, eliminate them. If you die, think of this: it is your family who will suffer. You need to find your song, the one that makes you move permanently in the direction of your goals and gives vision to your life. We all have a unique song to sing no matter the circumstance. Find your unique individual music and make it positive! It will improve your self-image, and it will be a call to action. All people have a natural way of relating and creating, and when you find yours, you will fulfill your dreams. You need to take control over your own life; no one will do it for you. "I just can't do it" is not acceptable. Visualize a life you would like to live and work toward it every day, even if you are only making small changes.

The changes will stimulate your immune system and your subconscious mind, and visualizing it will make it much more likely to happen. We can keep on doing the same things and expect different results, but that is just insanity.

When you have discovered your purpose, immediately begin to create momentum. Write down your purpose or goal frequently, and then do something daily to work toward this goal with some positive action. Set three-month, six-month, and one-year goals, and have a little celebration when you achieve each goal. Helping others may be the most motivating thing you can do; it sure works for me. Spirituality and religion create purpose for many people. Senseful purpose is the food on which our souls can thrive. Your age does not matter—use me as an example. We all need something to strive toward, so we can design our own inspiration. This will be different for different people. The secret to living is to create a meaningful purpose. The first step to creating any change is to decide what you want, not what you don't want. That is what will create a purpose in your life. Twenty percent of change is to know how to create it; and if you have opposition to change, you need to know why you're doing it. Dr. Rick Warren, famous evangelist, affirms that purpose is not a list of goals. Goals are temporary; purposes are eternal. It is a statement that points the direction of your life. He would say that if you tie your direction to your spiritual leader, whether that be God, Mohamed, Jesus, or a spirit or energy of the universe, it is much more likely to happen. Writing down your purposes forces you to think specifically about the path of your life, and knowing which way you are headed will keep you on solid ground. An intelligent person knows the direction he is going, but a fool starts going off in many different directions. Find out what your purpose is and start working on it today.

Genes

THE DEMONSTRATION OF OUR DNA helix by Dr. Watson and Dr. Crick in 1954 started the revolution of unraveling our genetic code. Our DNA is the future—. Many of our genes don't express themselves till later.

Genes play a role in longevity, just as they do in health and disease. It seems perhaps they only represent about 25 percent of our longevity.

Genes can be greatly influenced by what we do, what we eat, how much stress we endure, and how much we exercise.

We have about thirty thousand genes that are interdependent upon some interaction with the environment before they express themselves. Take the "thrifty gene" that many Africans, South Americans, Micronesians, and Japanese have that expresses itself only when they eat the wrong food. Africans who follow a vegetarian diet don't have the American diseases produced by the mad, sad, toxic way of eating.

We can turn our genes on and off depending on what we do; they are plastic. They also work together with other genes. Genes respond to hundreds of outside cues that switch them on and off.

Some genes are turned on and off by the nutrient density of foods. Foods of color have twenty thousand phytochemicals in them, they are enzymes that make it happen.

Genes knock on the door, but what you do unlocks it. Genes are not necessarily your future.

A Dr. Sinclair from Harvard Medical School has investigated a set of genes called the "sirtuin" genes, which are considered to be major influences on how long we live. When you modulate these genes, they turn on or turn off different metabolic pathways that are designed to promote longevity and health.

Dr. Sinclair's team has discovered that this gene can be affected by food restriction.

Studies on rats have proven if you restrict their food one third, they live 50 percent longer. That has been reproduced in many other living things except humans. However, there are some humans voluntarily practicing caloric restriction. I myself do not recommend caloric restriction, but I do recommend eating a nutritionally highly dense diet. However, if calorie restriction works in a lot of living things, I suspect it would have a greater effect also in humans. Let's face it: if you are very thin, you're not going to get many diseases and probably live a long life.

The specific genes involved are SIRT1. Dr. Sinclair published a now-famous paper reporting that plant compounds known as polyphenols could activate the human SIRT gene. As you might expect, pharmaceutical companies are now trying to exploit this potential.

Things we eat that manifest as oxidation, inflammation, and glycation will affect our longevity more generally than the genes we carry at birth, especially with the other twenty or so recommendations listed on the Longevity Mind-Body Index.

Telomeres are your future

TELOMERES SEQUENCES ARE AT THE ends of chromosomes. Chromosomes are in every one of your seventy trillion body cells. Written in the alphabet of the genes, telomeres do not contain the codes for proteins. Your chromosomes carry the code to make all the proteins in your body. So telomeres are not themselves genes, but neither are they meaningless junk. Instead, these repetitive sequences protect the ends of the chromosome from damage, including death.

When a cell divides, enzyme molecules copy the chromosomes. These molecules faithfully transcribe the genetic information on each chromosome, producing mere images of both of the two original strands. The enzyme molecules that do the duplicating are not able to completely reproduce the tips of the chromosomes, much as a tape recorder cannot play the last centimeters of a tape in a cassette. As a result, the duplicate chromosome is necessarily slightly shorter than the original, missing a small amount of the original telomeres sequence. The missing DNA does not measurably affect cellular functioning until enough subdivisions have occurred and the telomeres on at least one of the chromosomes in the cell becomes critically short.

Cells with critically short telomeres stop the duplication process of genes. They also become unresponsive to triggers that would normally stimulate them to divide. Though these growth-arrest chromosomes can live on in the body for years, once they have reached this state, they do not under normal circumstances replicate themselves. They are said to have reached their "Hayflick limit," named for the discoverer of the arrested state. Thus you can see eventually we reach a limit of the ability to divide, and the cells die—thus, there is a theory of aging.

There are a number of mechanisms in nature that counteract the natural tendency of telomeres erosion over time. Vertebrates, including mammals, use a remarkable enzyme called "telomerase." This hybrid molecule—part protein, part RNA—is capable of slowing telomere erosion, halting erosion altogether, or lengthening telomeres beyond those in the parent cell. The genes that produce telomerase are found in every potentially replicating cell in the body, including cells at their "Hayflick limits," but the genes that produce telomerase are inactive in the great majority of us for the vast bulk of our lives.

Telomeres are the major theory of aging at this time. When the age of reproduction typically begins in the species, individual animals decline in overall efficiency, and the vulnerability to injury and illness increases. The technical term for this decline is "senescence," though in common parlance the process is less precisely termed "aging."

Though the connection is still controversial, many researchers believe that the senescence decline observed in mammals is the result of an ever-increasing percentage of cells across the body reaching their "Hayflick" limits. At best, telomere erosion and "Hayflick" limits could account for most of the decline in efficiency and increases in vulnerability that characterize the aging of sexually mature mammals.

The evidence supporting this perspective has grown substantially in the last two years of research. Further, the discovery that several diseases that produce syndromes of apparently acceler-ated aging in humans, Hutchison-Guilford progeria and Werner's syndrome, now have been linked to telomere-system defects, strongly suggesting that this mechanism is fundamental to the explanation of aging in humans.

If the erosion of telomeres that accompanies cell division causes senescence, and if a cell is capable of producing an enzyme that can halt or reverse the process, why is the gene turned off in most tissues for most of our lives? Will everlasting youth be as simple as turning the gene back on all over the body?

Unfortunately, there's a very good reason to think that turn-ing telomerase back on across the body would be a disastrous mistake. Telomeres and telomerase, it turns out, are players in another active area of study, cancer. One of the most striking discoveries has been that cancer is rarely if ever the result of a single mutation. Generally, several complementary mutations must occur in the same cell to produce an ever-growing tumor. One of the most striking features that distinguish the majority of tumors and cancers from the normal tissue is that they arise as a product of the enzyme telomerase. Without telomerase, the cells in a tumor would quickly divide so may times that telomeres become critically short. Cell division would be arrested as cells run up against their Hayflick limits, and the small growth would likely go unnoticed. You can see the problem if we decide to extend life forever by fooling with nature.

The telomere is a region of repetitive DNA at the end of each chromosome, which protects the end of the chromosome from deterioration. Its name is derived from the Greek noun "telos" and "meros." The telomerases at the end of chromosomes allow for the shortening of chromosome ends, which necessarily occurs during chromosome replication.

PROVERBS 3:2

For length of days and years of life and peace they will add to you.

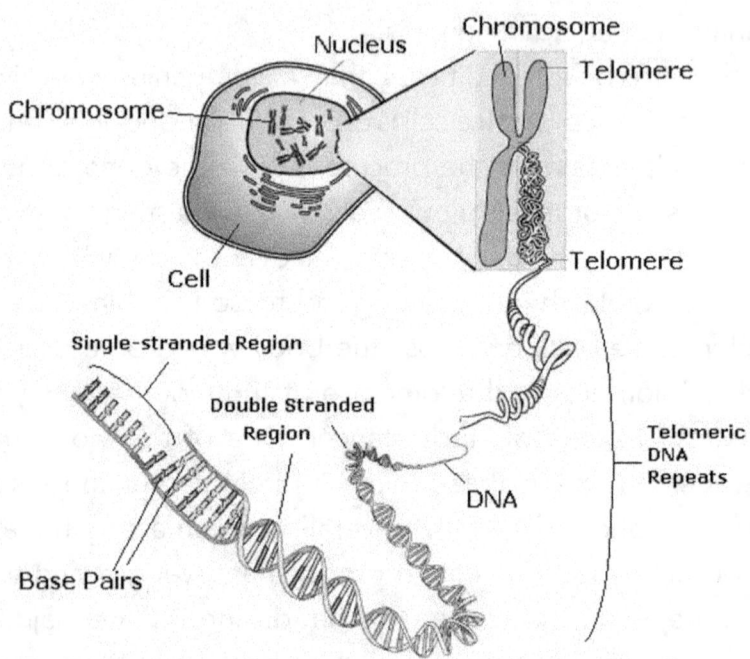

Proper Eating

THE LOW-CARBOHYDRATE CRAZE AND ENSUING widespread carbophobia changed the way Americans looked at the most fat-burning, satiating, and nutrient-dense food group: carbohydrates. Starchy carbohydrates like potatoes, corn, peas, whole-wheat pasta, multi-grain bread, kasha, and brown rice (plus many other whole grains, fruits, legumes, and vegetables) are an ancient food group—the same foods that our ancestors ate for thousands and thousands of years. Common sense and modern medical science beg us to rethink our aversion to carbohydrates, but many Americans continue to tell themselves that eating a twelve-ounce slab of prime rib is healthier than eating a baked potato.

Our bodies rely on two broad categories of chemicals on a regular basis: macronutrients, substances that we need to consume in larger quantities, and micronutrients, substances that we need in smaller amounts. Three major classes of macronutrients are essential to our health and well-being: carbohydrates, fats, and proteins. Carbohydrates are the body's first choice for fuel and the only nutrient that can effectively get to the brain and nervous system.

The commercial genius of the high-protein, low-carbohydrate diet was that it told Americans they could maintain their love of cheeseburgers, steak, bacon, and eggs and still lose weight. It was a devilish deal for the price of later complications such as hypertension, stroke, and clogged coronary arteries. Another reason why low-carbohydrate diets are popular, despite all the long-term health costs, is that they fit the American conspiracy mindset. Who wouldn't like to believe that thousands of scientific studies correlating the consumption of meat and dairy products with chronic disease were a big, fat lie?

Complex vs. Simple Carbohydrates

CARBOHYDRATES ARE NOT ALL THE same. The *amount* of carbohydrates in our diet doesn't affect us as much as the *quality* of those carbohydrates because our bodies metabolize *simple* and *complex* carbohydrates at different rates. Processing robs complex carbohydrates of key nutrients and fat-burning starch and turns them into simple carbohydrates, short chains of sugar molecules. Complex carbohydrates in fresh foods such as cantaloupes, lentils, and winter squash are made of long chains of sugar molecules and starch that will line the digestive tract and bind with water and cholesterol, leaving you full for much longer periods of time and even removing cholesterol from your bloodstream. High-fat, high-caloric protein foods such as chicken, beef, or cheese add cholesterol.

The best news is that we lose about 25 percent of the calories from Brussels sprouts, broccoli, Navy beans, oranges, and other complex carbohydrates in the energy spent during metabolism. We lose only 10 percent of the calories from simple carbohydrates during metabolism. The other 90 percent will end up as stored fat on our hips and bellies. Green and yellow vegetables, oatmeal, black beans, and other complex carbohydrates increase the thermic effect of food (TEF). They turn up our internal furnace, burning calories as heat and energy rather than converting them into fat. Even if we eat an excessive amount of carbohydrates, we will burn more calories in the energy spent converting them into glycogen, a high-octane reserve fuel stored in our liver, kidneys, and muscles.

The bulky fiber and starch in vegetables, (resistant starch), whole grains, legumes, and fruits take more energy to digest and break down into the bloodstream, prolonging the digestive process and increasing the resting metabolic rate (RMR). The energy expended at rest, our RMR, supports the work of our vital organs, such as the brain, heart, and lungs. A faster RMR means that more calories will be burned at rest—the easy way to lose weight.

At the molecular level, carbohydrates, fats, and protein have varying effects on our bodies. The conversion of complex carbohydrates to fat cells is a rare event. Even if we overeat nature's calorie burners, we'll still lose 25 percent of the calories in the energy spent during metabolism and another 20 percent of the calories in the energy spent to convert them to glycogen. But eating calories from simple carbohydrates versus complex carbohydrate calories will make you eat more calories.

SECRET: *All carbohydrates are not alike. Starchy complex carbohydrates quell hunger and turn up our internal furnace, burning calories as heat and energy. High-sugar, high-fat simple carbohydrates increase hunger, food addictions, and cravings.*

Disease-Fighting Fiber

Western Diseases

THE SECOND BIG ADVANTAGE OF starchy foods was discovered by the "Father of the Fiber Revolution," Dennis Burkitt, MD, who correlated our modern SAD diet of meat and processed foods and fewer fruits, whole grains, and vegetables with Western diseases: obesity, diabetes, vascular disease, and cancer. The Asians and Africans Dr. Burkitt studied ate a more traditional, fiber-rich diet of cassava, yams, millet, beans, whole-grain rice, starchy fruits, and green vegetables, and they enjoyed much lower rates of the diseases that plague our nation.

Root vegetables such as carrots and rutabaga and unprocessed cereals such as corn, barley, and steel-cut oats are more examples of fiber-rich carbohydrates. In Dr. Campbell's China study, starchy whole foods made up 90 percent of the traditional diet eaten by the disease-free Chinese. The average cholesterol level of the Chinese in the study was only 127 mg/dl—close to 100 points below the American average of 215 mg/dl.[1]

Late nineteenth-century inventions in wheat farming and flour milling marked a turning point in the American diet, forever changing our basic food staples such as breadstuffs. Revolutionary steel and porcelain grinders in flourmills began to convert wheat, corn, and other grains into superfine flour, eliminating two of the most nutrient-dense components of whole grains. The grinding removed the germ and the bran (the outer husk) from the wheat kernel, and then it crushed the inner kernel into flour. Flourmills were an important part of rural communities across the country.

Fiber controls the rate of digestion, has complex physiological effects on the digestive system and brain, and offers a variety of benefits such as lowering cholesterol, absorbing fat, and reducing the risk of colon cancer. Fiber is the only dietary factor that has convincing evidence showing a protective effect against weight gain and obesity.[2]

SECRET: *The same starchy carbohydrates that prevent disease and premature death can stop and even reverse disease.*

As fiber passes through the digestive tract, it absorbs minerals and eliminates fat, cholesterol, and cancer-causing toxins. Up to a third of fibrous, starchy complex carbohydrates are excreted by your body as waste. They *resist* digestion and provide few calories. Most simple carbohydrates like cake, cookies, and white bread are broken down into sugars that your body rapidly absorbs and stores as fat.

When "resistant starch" reaches the small intestine, bacteria use it as fuel, a process called fermentation, which protects colon cells from cancer. The starch travels undigested all the way through the small intestine. You literally *waste* more of the calories from starchy complex carbohydrates. Another benefit is that fiber and resistant starch help promote insulin sensitivity.

SECRET: *The "resistant starch" in complex carbohydrates absorbs fat and cholesterol, and it defies digestion while providing few calories and the feeling of fullness.*

The new refined flour could last longer and pack a better taste punch: as soon as the flour mixes with our saliva, it turns into sugar and raises insulin levels. A higher level of insulin in your blood means that your body will burn more blood sugar, giving you a nice jolt of energy but little else. Cells burn sugars preferentially. An hour or so after the Wonder Bread is gone, not only will your energy level plummet, your gut and brain will stimulate your appetite again. And off to the refrigerator you'll go. Insulin is one of the key hormones involved in appetite. Our obesity epidemic is in part an epidemic of *hyperinsulinemia*. Even those diet soft drinks that we consume trick our bodies and brains into stimulating our appetite. To avoid feeling tired and hungry all the time, skip the soft drinks and simple carbs and choose foods that are rich in fiber.

Simple carbohydrates are found in most commercial white breads, white rice, pretzels, french fries, beer, and in all the varieties of potato chips, soft drinks, baked goods, and candy bars. In our SAD diet, simple carbohydrates contribute about half of all calories and very few nutrients. Our bodies can break down simple carbohydrates quickly, resulting in an addicting but short-lived sugar high. The greater number of simple carbohydrates in your diet, the higher the "glycemic load," or spike in blood sugar, will be. As sugar levels in the blood rise, so does insulin. Surges of insulin push the body to store the excess sugar as fat. Studies show that chronic surges in insulin lead to chronic inflammation, weight gain, type 2 diabetes, and high cholesterol.[3] High-glycemic foods actually decrease the "good" HDL cholesterol that protects our arteries.

Unlucky Charms

HUNGER AND SATIETY ARE NOT the only reasons we start and stop eating. Researchers in the burgeoning field of food psychology have pinpointed a complex web of cues in the modern environment that all but overwhelm our adaptive systems: colors, presentation, portions, and food packaging. Parents can marvel at the multitude of cereal brands that promulgate the colorful, overcrowded cereal aisle. Lucky Charms, the most popular children's breakfast cereal on the market, boasts *Whole Grains* on the front of the box. But the amount of simple sugars found in one cup of the breakfast cereal cancels any nutritional value of the grains. Refined carbs offer a sweet taste and a short-lived surge of energy that can be very addicting, especially for young children. Simple carbs are sugars. Limit your total consumption of sugar to 10 percent or less of your daily calories to prevent the effects of insulin resistance.

Refined grains, such as white flour and white rice, have been processed, which removes nutrients and fiber. Unrefined grains still contain these vitamins and minerals and are rich in fiber, which helps your digestive system work well. Fiber also helps you feel full, so you're less likely to overeat. That explains why a bowl of oatmeal fills you up better than sugary cereal, which has the same number of calories as the oatmeal.

Best of all, whole grains help prevent vascular disease. In the Iowa Women's Health Study of thirty-four thousand women, those who ate at least one serving of whole grains each day had a 30 to 40 percent lower risk of vascular disease than women who ate no whole grains.[4]

SECRET: *Refined carbohydrates reduce the "good" HDL cholesterol and increase insulin levels, triglycerides, blood pressure, and fat stores—proven culprits in the development of inflammation, obesity, diabetes, and vascular disease.*

Be Wary of Breads with a Fake Tan

CONSUMERS SHOULD BE WARY OF deceptive advertising when it comes to whole grains. Manufacturers advertise many cereals, breads, crackers, pretzels, and even pasta products as "Whole Grain," but in reality these products are primarily made of white flour, sugar, chemicals, and additives, including caramel coloring. Coarsely ground grains curtail our appetite better and provide disease-fighting nutrients. Check the ingredients on the label to watch out for "Whole Grain" products with a fake tan. If multi-grains, wheat, corn, rice, bulgur, millet, oats, or another grain aren't listed within the first two ingredients, move on to the next loaf.

Maximizing Nutrients

FRESHNESS, PREPARATION, AND COOKING MAKE a difference in maximizing the amount of nutrients you receive from unprocessed carbohydrates. Slightly green bananas have more resistant starch and less sugar than ripened bananas. If you cool cooked starches, such as potatoes and whole-wheat pasta, you can increase the amount of resistant starch in the food. Pasta should be cooked "al dente" (slightly firm). The more you cook pasta, the faster it is broken down into sugar. Cooking carrots releases more nutrients than if you would eat the vegetable raw. But overcooking vegetables can ruin a perfectly good source of disease-fighting nutrients. Overcooking vegetables reduces the amount of phytochemicals, vitamins, and other nutrients that enter our body.

Many people think that complex carbohydrates such as potatoes are fattening. A baked potato has almost no fat and no cholesterol and is high in fiber, but if you add butter and sour cream, you're transforming an ideal food into one very high in fat and cholesterol. The trick is to eat a small potato and dress up it without adding fats.

Choose Foods
that Burn Fat

UNDERSTANDING AND TAKING ADVANTAGE OF how your body uses and stores energy is the key to good health and maximum weight loss. Your cells metabolize energy or calories from protein, carbohydrates, and fats. Calories "in" are not calories "out." It takes more calories to digest and metabolize the starch and nutrients in complex carbohydrates. It takes much less energy or calories to metabolize fats and simple sugars. Your body stores complex carbohydrates within cells as glycogen, a nutrient that the body can easily and rapidly convert to energy.

Foods that promote weight loss are high in complex carbohydrates. Your body requires much more energy to break down and digest their critical nutrients. When you eat high complex carbohydrate foods such as whole grains, fruits, and vegetables, your body increases your metabolism, which in turn promotes weight loss. In fact, you'll lose 45 percent of the calories from complex carbohydrates during digestion alone. Oftentimes these foods have fewer calories than it takes the body to process and use them. The increase in metabolism can burn excess body fat. Nutritious foods promote weight loss!

SECRET: *Foods that promote weight loss are high in complex carbohydrates, which take more energy (calories) to break down. Your metabolism speeds up to process the critical nutrients of these foods. A faster metabolism can burn excess body fat.*

Complex Carbohydrates on the Brain

FOOD ALSO AFFECTS OUR BRAIN chemistry, for better or worse. Tryptophan is one of the essential amino acids that our brain uses to synthesize serotonin, a powerful neurotransmitter. Serotonin improves mood, reduces appetite, and induces sleep, among other things. High-protein foods such as beef, turkey, or fish contain high levels of tryptophan, but they also have large quantities of the other amino acids that compete with tryptophan to reach the brain. Protein actually has a negative effect on tryptophan and serotonin levels. Studies have shown that women on a high-protein diet tend to have trouble sleeping; this may be in part due to the reduction in serotonin.

According to research by Drs. Richard and Judith Wurtman of the Massachusetts Institute of Technology, insulin drives long-chained amino acids out of blood circulation and into tissues and organs. Eating lots of low-protein, high-carbohydrate starches, vegetables, and fruits raises insulin, which encourages amino acids to leave blood circulation, with the result that more tryptophan can enter the brain. When the supply of tryptophan increases, serotonin increases, and appetite decreases. And that is why complex carbohydrates turn off the appetite and create a feeling of satisfaction.

SECRET: *Consumption of complex carbohydrates helps the brain produce higher levels of serotonin, which reduces your appetite and increases your feeling of well-being.*

Getting Over Carbophobia

WHEN THE TRILLION-DOLLAR FOOD INDUSTRY throws its marketing weight behind a dieting fad, our perception of a certain type of food can change for better or for worse. In the heyday of the Atkins Diet, many doctors recommended a low-fat, high-carbohydrate diet to their patients but didn't distinguish between simple or complex carbohydrates. The Institute of Medicine, the unit of the National Academies that sets our recommended daily intake values for nutrients, has set 130 grams of complex carbohydrates as the recommended minimum daily intake for adults and children.

Animal-based products such as meat, dairy, and eggs—the foods richest in artery-clogging cholesterol—are deficient in fiber. Beef, fish, and poultry also decrease our serotonin levels. The sugar rush you crave after the average high protein, high-fat American meal is your body's attempt to raise serotonin levels and improve your mood.

Complex carbohydrates fuel our brains. As we chew food, our saliva releases a digestive enzyme called alpha amylase that is crucial for breaking down starch into glucose. Our brain runs on glucose. Primates and other animals with smaller brains lack the genetic code to manufacturer the enzyme.

Evolutionary scientists theorize that our unique ability to digest starchy carrots, onions, and potatoes gave our ancestors enough glucose to develop large brains over time. And when our body metabolizes starch, the resulting by-products, carbon dioxide and water, are easily eliminated from the body. In contrast, animal protein requires much more effort to convert to energy, and its by-product, nitrogen, converts to ammonia and urea, both of which can be harmful, especially to the vascular system, kidneys, and liver. Our body handles starchy carbohydrates more efficiently, leaving us feeling more alert, energized, and satisfied.

Starch: Nature's Statin

STARCHY COMPLEX CARBOHYDRATES, VEGETABLES, LEGUMES, whole grains, and fruit offer fiber, antioxidants, and minerals. Fiber blocks the synthesis of cholesterol, slows down glucose absorption, and controls the rate of digestion. Many carbohydrates even resist digestion. They're our best weapon against the trio of insulin resistance, obesity, and vascular disease.

The simple carbohydrates in white pasta, white bread, and other refined foods are not only stripped of disease-fighting nutrients and fiber, they stimulate our pancreas to produce insulin. If we eat too many simple carbohydrates, our body begins to store the excess glucose as fat. Overindulging on simple carbohydrates can lead to insulin resistance and obesity.

Best of all, unprocessed carbohydrates improve our mood and provide sustained energy. The strongest evidence for a way of eating that prolongs lifespan favors starchy, complex carbohydrates—nature's miracle fat-burners and nutritional winners.

PSALM 21:4
He asked life of you; you gave it to him, length of days forever and ever.

Great Immunity -
"The Gold"

THE ARMY, NAVY, AIR FORCE, and marines (the immune system) that defend our health will determine our lifespan. Dr. Joel Fuhrman wrote another great book, *Super Immunity*, which was recently published, and it really is the gold of longevity and health teaching. I read a pre-published copy twice, and the publisher asked me to write a few words about it. I think that unless you fall out of an airplane, if you follow what is recommended, including the recipes in the back of the book, you have a 90% chance of living to be one hundred or better with a sound mind. It is all about a nutrient-dense way of eating in which you eat the right macro and micro nutrients, vitamins, and minerals; the right complex carbohydrates; 100 percent whole grains; proteins; fats; and phytochemicals. That creates a strong immune system, a system that prevents vascular disease, heart attacks, strokes, cancer, infections, autoimmune disease, etc.

The China Study, by Colin Campbell, proved that certain foods could provide health promotion and disease protection benefits. The study was done a few decades ago, but a lot of this information has been known for thousands of years. Natural plants are complex packages of biologically active compounds. The term "phytochemicals," which means "of plant chemicals," represents the thousands of plant source compounds that have profound effects on human health and immunity. Scientific discoveries have proven that the phytochemicals run the machinery of metabolism; they are the co-enzymes that run the chemical reactions of our body. Our food, in other words, helps determine resistance to disease and increases our longevity. The benefits of good eating habits have been largely ignored by 80 percent of the American people, resulting in a lot of diseases, poor health, and tremendous cost. Koreans, Japanese, Micronesians, South Americans, and Africans are being devastated by the sad, mad, toxic diet of fat, salt, and sugar. The human body can take advantage of the complex biochemical compounds found in plants that we can use to keep a normal weight, prevent illness, and heal previously damaged cells. We have stopped our overemphasis on vitamins and minerals and started paying attention to the defense and repair mechanism of our body's twenty-five thousand phytochemicals. The phytochemicals are bioactive, plant-derived chemical compounds important for the growth and survival of the planet. The human immune system evolved dependent on the phytochemicals for its optimal functioning. The plants use these phytochemicals to defend themselves against their enemies—funguses, viruses, bacteria, and animals.

Superior nutrition is the secret of the "superior immunity" that Dr. Joel Fuhrman writes about. You don't have to be a genius to realize that. There is great synergism of the human immune system and the phytochemicals of our plants.

Animals and plants have developed a fragile, interconnected, and symbiotic relationship on earth. Now human beings rely on plants for health and survival.

We are what we eat. We are made from what we eat. Fat, salt, and sugar are not going to do it for you. That's what Americans eat 80 percent of the time, and look at their obesity rate—65 percent. One third of children are overweight. When we cultivate nutritional deficiencies in our body over long periods of time, especially in our formative years, it creates a lot of cellular damage, resulting in serious illnesses late in life. Advancements in nutritional sciences have created an opportunity for great health and longevity, preventing disease including cancer, heart attacks, and strokes, which are well known in vegetarian societies. The chemical compounds found in vegetables, beans, berries, and fruits, when combined with nuts, seeds, mushrooms, and onions, fuel the miraculous self-healing and self-protective properties already built into the human genome. The American diet is a disaster of processed foods and animal products, which represent 85 percent of a mad, sad diet and are very low in nutrients, natural vegetables, and phytochemicals, and as a result of marketing are dramatically deficient in plant-derived, disease-fighting chemicals. We consume less than 10 percent of our foods from unrefined foods. Ninety percent of our food has been stripped of healthy fiber. We are not eating enough fruits, beans, seeds, and vegetables. We are missing the beneficial antioxidants and phytochemicals that repair the body and prevent disease. The carotene family, alpha and beta, lutein, zeayanthin, lycopene, flavonoids, alpha-lipoic acid, quercetin, anthcyanins, ligans, and pectins, etc. are among the great chemicals that can heal us and prevent cancer and numerous inflammatory diseases, and they are found in the vegetables and beans we eat. Since neither processed foods nor animal products contain a significant load of antioxidant nutrients and phytochemicals, the modern diet is dramatically disease prone.

Antioxidants are vitamins, minerals, and phytochemicals that aid the body in removing free radicals, which cause diseases that kill us. The vast majority of antioxidants are available to the body through fruits, vegetables, and other natural plants. Oxidative damage occurs when free radical activity in the body increases and free radicals burst out of their cellular compartments to affect broader regions of the cells. Vegetables are so rich in anti-oxidant chemical compounds that eating a vegetarian, vegan, or nutritarian diet is an easy way to increase antioxidant capacity. Foods with great amounts of phytochemicals are cabbage, red peppers, carrots, green peppers, tomatoes, onions, broccoli, peas, squash, and mushrooms. A phytochemical-deficient diet is responsible for a weak immune system, resulting in disease and death at a young age. Populations with much higher amounts of vegetables in their diet have 50 to 70 percent lower rates of cancer and inflammatory diseases. The longest-living populations throughout history are the ones with a high intake of vegetables in their diet. Dr. Joel Fuhrman says that the phytochemicals are the most important discovery in human nutrition over the last fifty years. The concentration of phytochemicals is often highlighted by vibrant colors of black, blue, red, green, and orange—except maybe for the very healthy mushrooms.

The benefits of phytochemicals are:
- Detoxifying enzymes
- Controlling the production of free radicals
- Deactivation and detoxification of cancer-producing agents
- Protecting cell structure from damage by toxins
- Fueling mechanisms to repair damaged DNA
- Introducing beneficial antifungal, antibacterial, and anti-viral effects

- Inhibiting the function of damaged or genetically altered DNA
- Improving immune cells function
- Producing great disease-fighting antibodies, preventing cancer

THE WAR ON CANCER

Our cancer rates exploded between 1935-2005. There has been an increasing rate every year for seventy years. We've had an explosion of immune system dependent diseases, allergies, autoimmune disease, and cancer.

Cruciferous vegetables are great anticancer agents. Green vegetables such as kale, cabbage, broccoli, cauliflower, and turnips are called cruciferous vegetables because as a flower, they have four petals like a cross. Cruciferous vegetables have a unique chemical composition. They make a sulfur-containing compound, where the cells are programmed to release ITC's, an array of compounds with proven powerful immune-boosting effects in anticancer activity. Eating cruciferous vegetables, chewing them and breaking the cellular structure, decreases cancer rates dramatically. Consuming mushrooms regularly is associated with significant decrease in the risk of breast cancer. Frequent consumption of mushrooms can decrease the incidence of breast cancer 60 to 70 percent. So what's the solution? Dr. Furman has a great formula: $H=N/C$. Health expectancy equals nutrient density divided by calories. There is our destiny.

To slow the aging process, we need to eat a nutrient-dense diet. Vegetables, beans, and fruits, essentially all you can eat. Counting calories or portion control is not needed if you eat nutrient-dense foods.

Dr. Furman's diet in his book *Eat to Live*:
- Vegetable based
- Lots of fruits, beans
- Seeds and nuts
- Oil used sparingly
- Animal products zero to three times a week

The Standard American diet:
- Grain-based
- Lots of dairy and meat
- Lots of oil
- Major animal products
- Animal products five to seven times a week
- Focus on nutrient-poor calories

The Gold

"Resistant starches" means starches with a lot of fiber. The starchy foods will not be all absorbed because of high fiber content. At least 30 to 40 percent of calories are lost in metabolism. They never enter the bloodstream. The starch from a baked potato will have a high absorption rate because of lack of fiber. Calories in and calories out—the original concept was incorrect. Beans promote a sensation of fullness. They improve insulin sensitivity, decreasing diabetes. Beans promote good bacteria once the bowel has adjusted. Beans have in them also a lot of good essential fatty acids, which you need. The carbohydrates in them have a lot of fiber and will not be all absorbed, and you can eat a lot of them because of that.

- Black beans – 63 percent fiber
- Red kidney beans – 56 percent fiber

- Navy beans – 52 percent fiber
- Lentils – 47 percent fiber
- Split peas – 38 percent fiber
- Corn – 32 percent fiber

The nutritionally highly dense diet will enhance cellular repair mechanisms and reverse disease. That is why the way of eating that that Dr. Dean Ornish recommends for preventing, stopping, and reversing heart disease works. He essentially teaches the same thing that Dr. Furman and I teach. This way of eating reduces the inflammatory response, suppresses genetic alterations, decreases free radical activity, slows the metabolic rate, enhances DNA repair, and removes toxins.

WHAT IS A NUTRITARIAN?

A nutritarian is a person whose food choices are influenced by nutritional quality. It is a person who strives for more micronutrients per calorie in the diet and who recognizes that food is a powerful disease fighter for an effective and therapeutic effect. Nuts and seeds are good for weight loss. They have a lot of fiber in them, and they carry a lot of good essential fatty acids. You should eat at least one ounce a day. A lot of people get away with two ounces because it tremendously decreases the appetite.

How do you prevent, stop, and reverse vascular disease and diabetes?

- Eat at least 50 g of fiber daily.
- Eat a 20 percent fat diet—fat from seeds, nuts, and vegetables.
- Eat sufficient omega-3—your essential fatty acids.

- Eat a high-phytochemical and antioxidant diet.
- Eat low-glycemic index foods.
- Eat low-calorie, dense foods.
- Limit animal products to two to three servings a week.

IGF

High levels of the hormone IGF reduces longevity and leads to cancer. Low levels lead to increased lifespan and decrease inflammation, decrease oxidative damage, increase insulin sensitivity, and slow the aging process. The amount of meat we eat determines the IGF level. We have at least twenty major recommendations to live to be one hundred and be of sound mind. But what to eat by far will have the greatest effect. Your food selection is critical to your longevity.

Our Friends and Healthy Eating

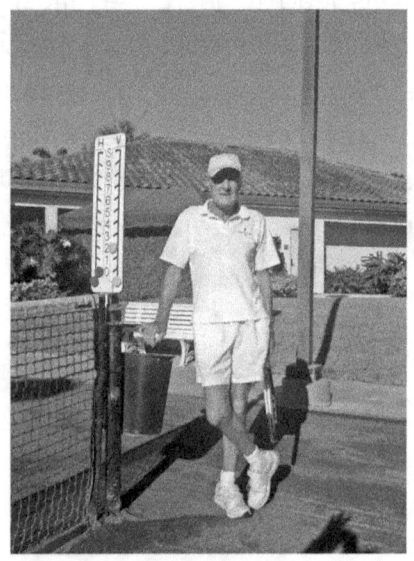

BEING HEALTHY CAN, AND SHOULD, be a way of life. Sure, we can break it down to healthy eating, exercise, weight control, and stress, but above all one must have the desire. To give up smoking is not just a question of being ostracized or seeing the health hazards. Some people see those and never stop smoking. You really have to have the desire and self-discipline to do it. The same applies to all aspects of Aristotle's view of the good life. To address the healthy eating part of the "good life" plan means taking deliberate steps to investigate and understand what is fundamentally essential for the body and mind to be sustained and grow. Basically, I believe in using in my diet as many natural and unprocessed foods as possible. Breakfast will consist of raw oats with soy or low fat milk or no milk at all, just water. Lunchtime is always fresh fruit and vegetables, usually consisting of a half cup of carrots plus either apple, mango, or melon. Dinner might be pasta with tomatoes, mushrooms, etc., or fish such as salmon and always with either yams or regular potatoes and a fresh vegetable such as broccoli, brussels sprouts, cauliflower, or snow peas.

I believe that it is also important to stress that the diet I have described is very economical. The food cost is approximately half of those with the normal fast and prepared food diets. You can buy a pound of oats for about a dollar, just a third of the cost of a prepared cereal.

I accompany this with regular exercise, consisting of either tennis or a forty-minute fast walk in the morning and then another walk, either late afternoon or in the evening after dinner. The result is a seventy-eight-year-old, 144-pound man who feels great.

Thank you Mike, my friend in Naples Florida.

Hypertension:
The Silent Killer

WE ALL NEED TO KNOW about blood pressure. Hypertension leads to strokes and heart disease and starts at a very young age, even as a teenager.

Millions of people are walking around with elevated blood pressure and don't know it, ticking time bombs. It causes terrific damage to the vasculature of the body, the plumbing that leads to the vital organs. Sudden heart attacks and strokes, even at a young age, are not that unusual in people who have had hypertension for a few years.

Certain ethnic and racial groups are particularly prone to hypertension, the degree of which is frankly not believable. When I was a resident of neurosurgery at the inner-city hospital at Georgetown University in Washington, DC, I operated on about two major brain hemorrhages a day secondary to rampant hypertension. You do not see this kind of hypertension in their grandparents who lived in Africa. In 1954 in Kenya, Africa, medical schools could hardly find a patient with a stroke or heart attack to show to the students. The population was eating a vegetarian diet and did not have the problems of the American African people. It's based on genetics, sodium sensitivity, and largely diet.

If you keep your blood pressure normal, you can avoid a lot of diseases. I was working out at the YMCA today, where I had established a wellness center in the inner city because of this problem. I spoke to a very muscular black gentleman, and we discussed his blood pressure. He had had a very significant problem, but working out four to five days a week returned his blood pressure to normal. He promised me that he would help do some teaching at my new wellness center in the inner city. It was a great day for me.

If you have hypertension and elevated cholesterol, I'd be amazed if you live to be a hundred, unfortunately. So we must educate ourselves, get our blood pressure checked, and act.

The medical community started realizing the impact of high blood pressure around 1972 and did not realize that chronic inflammatory factors from fat were at play—and they were at the end of the discussion. It's the inflammatory factors of fat that lead to vascular disease and hypertension.

At least one third of Americans age eighteen to sixty-five have at least mild hypertension. For Afro-Americans it's 50 percent, and one third are not being treated. If you combine that with a family history of hypertension, high cholesterol, high CRP and obesity, things get even worse statistically. There is increased risk of dementia with hypertension. The famous Farmington Heart Study from Massachusetts proved that point. The first symptom of hypertension may be an unexpected heart attack or stroke.

I'll be recommending a combination of many things—exercising to reach a normal BMI, a low-sodium diet, and some supplements to bring your blood pressure under control. It's a combination that adds up, and it can bring blood pressure almost to normal without medication most of the time. Your ideal blood pressure is 115/75. 160 and over is malignant hypertension and needs to be treated right away.

Hypertension is a silent killer, and symptoms are rare. That's why you to have it checked even at a young age, frequently. I suggest you buy a blood pressure monitor from your local pharmacy and check it frequently and keep a log. One abnormal reading does not do it. Headaches are rare with hypertension. Family history is important. Almost all type II diabetics have hypertension.

Hypertension generally develops slowly. But blood pressure is a force that drives your blood against the walls of the arteries and delivers it to your major organs. The heart beats only sixty to seventy times a minute. Systolic pressure, the top number, is the contraction of the heart; diastolic, the bottom number, is the relaxation.

Blood pressure is controlled by three basic methods.

First, there are pressure receptors in various organs that send electrical impulses or chemicals to the heart. Second, the kidneys have receptors for long-term adjustments and work through chemicals—the renin-angiotensin system. Third, aldostrone, a hormone from the adrenal gland, responds to increased levels of angiotensin and potassium. Aldosterone has an effect on potassium and sodium in the body, which affect your blood pressure.

Blood pressure, smoking, inflammation, and cholesterol are the four forces of cardiovascular disease. Also they can be markers of hypertension. In the general white population, 20 percent have hypertension. This number is 31 percent in the African American population, 19 percent in the Hispanic population, and 60 percent in the Asian population. We have 7.2 million heart attacks per year and 5.5 million strokes. The majority of these people have high blood pressure. African Americans are more sodium sensitive than whites; this is probably based on evolution. It is my experience that obesity, diabetes, hypertension, heart attacks, and strokes are more common in the American African population. This is not so in Africa; the problem appears to be the diet. That's why I started a wellness center in the inner city, and my visit there today was heartwarming. I made many friends there who were willing to help me try to bring about changes.

Headaches, dizziness, and nosebleeds are not common symptoms of hypertension.

DEFINITION

Hypertension is high blood pressure. Blood pressure is the force of blood pushing against the walls of arteries as it flows through them. Arteries are the blood vessels that carry oxygenated blood from the heart to the body's tissues.

As blood flows through arteries, it pushes against the inside of the artery walls. The more pressure the blood exerts on the artery walls, the higher the blood pressure will be. The size of small arteries also affects blood pressure. When the muscular walls of arteries are relaxed, or dilated, the pressure of the blood flowing through them is lower than when the artery walls narrow, or constrict.

Blood pressure is highest when the heart beats to push blood out into the arteries. When the heart relaxes to fill with blood again, the pressure is at its lowest point. Blood pressure when the heart beats is called systolic pressure. Blood pressure when the heart is at rest is called diastolic pressure. When blood pressure is measured, the systolic pressure is stated first and the diastolic pressure second. Blood pressure is measured in millimeters of mercury (mm Hg). For example, if a person's systolic pressure is 120 and diastolic pressure is 80, it is written as 120/80 mm

Hg. The American Heart Association has long considered blood pressure less than 140 over 90 normal for adults. However, the National Heart, Lung, and Blood Institute in Bethesda, Maryland, released new clinical guidelines for blood pressure in 2003, lowering the standard normal readings. A normal reading was lowered to less than 120 over less than 80.

Hypertension is a major health problem, especially because it has no symptoms. Many people have hypertension without knowing it. In the United States, about 50 million people age sixty and older have high blood pressure. Hypertension is more common in men than women and in people over the age of sixty-five than in younger persons. More than half of all Americans over the age of sixty-five have hypertension. It also is more common in African-Americans than in white Americans.

Hypertension is serious because people with the condition have a higher risk for heart disease and other medical problems than people with normal blood pressure. Serious complications can be avoided by getting regular blood pressure checks and treating hypertension as soon as it is diagnosed.

People over fifty with hypertension have a high rate of heart attacks and strokes. The pre-hypertensive population is large. Checking your blood pressure is important. Multiple readings are so much more helpful than just one or two. Don't grab for a pill unless you're unable to change your lifestyle and bring it under control within a month or two.

Native Americans have the same problem of increased rate of hypertension, This is also true for Asians and Micronesians, especially those eating the mad, sad, toxic American diet. The people in Micronesia have a 90 percent hypertension rate as well as diabetes. You think they'll have a long life? Do you think you will live to be a hundred? I don't think so! They are not going to live a long life if they don't treat high blood pressure!

Hypertension in pregnancy is especially life threatening to the mother and the child, You should check your blood pressure daily if you're pregnant.

Blood Pressure and Diabetes

DR. ROBERT E. KOWALSKI WROTE a great book on blood pressure and cholesterol, he says "I consider every diabetic patient to be a heart patient." If you have type II diabetes, you have a 90 percent chance of having vascular disease, and 65 percent of diabetics will die from a heart attack.

Weight and Hypertension

WE HAVE AN INCREASED OBESITY rate in children now. Our type II diabetic rate is doubling every ten years, and two thirds of us are overweight. In Canada, 50 percent of men and women are overweight.

As you gain weight, blood pressure increases. Inflammatory factors in fat cause nasty disease, heart attacks, strokes, cancer, dementia, and autoimmune diseases. Your CRP, C reactive protein is a measure of the inflammation in your blood. This is an important test.

Your weight is best evaluated with the BMI and the waist/hip ratio. You can refer to BMI tables, which I've included in this book.

BMI less than 25 is good, over 30 is overweight, 35 is obese, and 40 is morbidly obese. Waist measurement for men should be 35 inches or less, 30 inches or less for women. You waist-hip ratio should be less than one.

I've written a book called *The Secret of the Nondiet*. It outlines four different ways of eating that eliminate type II diabetes in those of normal weight 90 percent of the time. I recommend you read it if you have a problem.

Basically it's a combination of vegetarian, vegan, flexitarian, and nutritarian ways of eating. It's not a diet, just nutritionally highly dense foods, essentially all-you-can-eat. Diets don't work.

I recommend exercise. Exercise is at least one third of weight control and makes you feel more energetic. I work out every day, and I must say it really makes me feel great.

A lot of us are stress eaters. Food is a drug. I recommend my book *The Psychology of Eating*. I think it's quite helpful.

I wrote five books on proper eating and call them "the magic five." I recommend you read them as they lead to good health and a long happy life.

If you see a potbelly on someone, odds are, unfortunately, that that person is chronically stressed out and uses food as a drug of choice. It's a difficult problem, but it can be conquered. Reading my chapter on stress could help you understand the nature of it. Let's face it: we all have stress. It's a war in the kitchen when I come home after a stressful day of neurosurgery. I've developed a system of dealing with it, but it sure doesn't work every time. Then again, I weigh 145 pounds, so it must be working, and frankly I am not perfect. None of us are.

I would now like to recommend some other holistic methods to get your blood pressure under control without expensive, risky medications. I recommend holistic methods of treating this condition for a few months, depending on the circumstances. Of course, if you have had a stroke or very high blood pressure, I would recommend medicine right away. We're talking about preventative methods and treatments!

The Condition of Your
Vascular Pipes

THE CONDITION OF YOUR VASCULATURE determines whether you will have a stroke, heart attack, neuropathy, blindness, or amputations, and it is determined in large part by your blood pressure.

The inner membrane of your vessel is called the endothelium. Researchers have found that this membrane releases a substance that improves the elasticity and flexibility of your blood vessels. The endothelial layer is very thin. They originally called the chemical EDRF, endothelial derived relaxing factor. Researchers finally discovered it to be a gas, nitric acid, and they received the Nobel Prize for that in 1998.

Thirty thousand scientific papers have been published on nitric acid since that time.

One of the building blocks of nitric acid is arginine. Blood pressure is greatly affected by the amount of nitric acid in the blood. Nitric acid, NA, relaxes the arteries and makes them more compliant, flexible so they can be dilated. Nitric acid also inhibits ACE, angiotensin converting enzyme, which raises blood pressure. As we age, nitric acid declines, so increasing nitric acid is part of our blood pressure fighting program.

Actually Dr. Robert Kowalski doesn't agree that our arteries harden as we get older. People following largely a vegetarian diet in other countries have not been found to develop hypertension, and the arteries remain quite compliant and soft. Causes of stiffening are smoking, sedentary lifestyle, diabetes, high cholesterol, hypertension, inflammation, and obesity.

Certain ethnic and racial groups have less nitric acid in their blood and therefore a higher rate of hypertension, such as the Asian and black population. When I was a resident neurosurgeon at Georgetown in Washington, DC, brain hemorrhage from hypertension in the black community was extremely common. The blood pressures I would see were well beyond comprehension because we did not have good medication at that time and dietary teaching was nonexistent. I'm talking about pressures of 300/200.

So what's the program of blood pressure control?

Ideal blood pressures should not be greater than 120/80. 120-139/80-89 is pre-hypertension. 140/90 is hypertension.

Pressure measuring devices should be as common as scales at home. Blood pressures should be checked frequently and recorded. One or two readings don't do it. You should check the blood pressure of your teenagers; obesity and blood pressure problems can start at any age. It foretells the future. If you're hypertensive at a young age and don't do anything about it, you will not live to be a hundred.

What's the program?
- Maintain a normal-weight BMI.
- Eat a nutritionally highly dense diet as described in the book *Secret of the Non-Diet for Adults* by Rudy Kachhman, MD.
- Exercise and lift light weights regularly.
- Practice stress control.

Supplements

1. Arginine
www.endure.com
2. Grape seed extract
www.polyphenolics.com
3. Lyc-Mato—a tomato extract
www.swansonorgins.com
4. Pine bark extract
wwwpycnogenal.com

A good discussion of the supplements is detailed in Dr. Robert Kowalski's book. Check with your doctor before taking them.

I would certainly recommend trying these very effective holistic methods for a couple months unless you are under an emergency situation. I would say 90 percent of people with hypertension can control it without medication if they follow the above recommendations. Certainly if you're in the hospital with a heart attack or stroke or brain hemorrhage, blood pressure medication would be required. Also, of course, if your blood pressure is out of sight, medication becomes necessary immediately. Always let your doctor know what you are doing. Then again, the majority of physicians do not recommend lifestyle changes up front. Unfortunately, that is from my experience. Good luck.

JOB 42:16

And after this Job lived 140 years, and saw his sons, and his sons' sons, four generations.

Exercise

LEARN TO DANCE—ONE OF THE secrets of motivating yourself to wellness. All types of dance are great. I'm speaking about the use of rhythm and movement to improve your longevity and intelligence. You have to use your mind to dance correctly. Ballroom dancing improves the mind and the body. Join a class and do this one or two days a week regularly.

So whenever you are moving in rhythm, whether or not music is playing, you can consider yourself to be dancing. The dances of walking, jogging, biking, swimming, hiking, and even golf or tennis are following a rhythm. Keeping in rhythm means the timing of the swing, shot after shot, so you develop consistency. I play a lot of tennis. I have all my life, and really it's a form of dancing.

The effect of exercise on the immune system has been scientifically proven. Scientists have found that exercise has a direct effect on our white blood cells, the main cells affecting our immunity. After a few months of exercise, the levels of immune activating nasty cytokines produced by white cells drop over 50 percent, while the levels of immune protective good cytokines rise about 35 percent, scientific studies have proven. Exercise is probably the single most effective way to lower inflammatory factors in the blood that cause cancer and vascular disease.

When physical activity is done through rhythm, it can be considered dance, a powerful way to get the most benefit from your exercise program. Pilates, for example, is an excellent way, as well as all other basic yoga activities. Chi-gong, tai chi, kundalini yoga, and dancing have the greatest effect on the inflammatory factors in your blood, the CRP (C-Reactive Protein) levels. Researchers have found greatly beneficial effects on anxiety and depression in people who performed exercises such as jogging, swimming, cycling, and walking. And music rehabilitation and physical therapy programs for Parkinson's disease patients also have been shown to improve outcomes when compared to standard physical exercises. Any rhythm to movement certainly increases the level of enjoyment and involvement in exercise classes. The addition of pumping rhythmic music to aerobic exercise classes encourages participation and increases satisfaction levels. Ask me and I will tell you—I own a wellness studio, and it works for our clients and me. Turning a standard exercise routine into a dance is more fun, less boring, and ensures that exercise is kept at their activity level.

Why does rhythmic exercise works so much better? RHYTHMIC contraction, alternating between flexion and extension, provides balance and strengthens both flexors and extensors equally. The nerve impulses that regulate muscle groups originate from signals in the brain and are transmitted along the spinal cord. The same neurotransmitter chemicals released by our brain and nerve endings are sensed by our immune system. When a brain is dancing, so is our immune system. Human life itself consists of rhythms; it's quite possible that the immune system responds to these rhythms.

Rhythm is an integral part of life and is as old as history. Look at the old religions, tribal dancing, Hinduism. Dancing is thought to be the Arum of the universe. In Hinduism, you've heard of the ancient cosmic dance of Shiva. The frequency and randomness of all such sounds are considered to hold healing powers, as is the vocalization "ohm." Apollo, the son of Zeus and the God of medicine, was known as a dancer. In Sparta, authorities required parents to instruct their children in the art of dancing, beginning at the age of five. Dancing is thought to be good for the body and overall health, as well as for the soul. In modern science, researchers have shown that music in rhythm produces measurable healing effects. Music has been proven to reduce stress and anxiety, as evidenced by multiple studies of heart patients who underwent catheterization and other unpleasant procedures. These patients' anxiety levels were significantly reduced when music was played during cardiac catheterization.

The brain uses a rhythm to heal. It is important to breathe in rhythm because it affects our immunity. Healers across many different cultures have employed dance to induce a trance as part of a healing ritual. The Chinese discipline known as tai chi, which originated more than eight centuries ago, is still used as a healing art. Tai chi creates a meditative state that is set to restore natural rhythms and balance in the mind and the body. When you combine movement with rhythm, you enjoy the double benefit of exercise and the meditative state; you lower the inflammatory factors in the blood. It is better when you have a bit of low-back pain to do some rhythmic movement. It's better than lying in bed or on the couch all day.

WHAT ACTION SHOULD YOU TAKE?

- Walking for thirty minutes every day, in rhythm
- Swimming
- Doing entry-level aerobics and advancing over time
- Ballroom dancing—I did it for two years with two Russian dancers.
- Biking
- Rowing
- Jogging
- Jumping rope
- Tap, hip-hop, square dancing
- Participating in competitive sports
- Practicing martial arts
- Getting a personal trainer
- Starting a weight-training program

Exercise Enhances
Your Brain and Longevity

WE NEED TO GO BACK into our evolutionary history to demonstrate the relationship between brain growth, increasing intelligence, and exercise.

To survive after forest life declined, we had to start running for our food, and our brain started growing. Two million years ago, Homo erectus had to leave those vending machines, the beautiful forests, to catch his food, sometimes traveling ten to twenty miles a day. Our more direct ancestors, Homo sapiens, had to run even farther. Now our ancestors had access to oceans and lakes and those beautiful omega-3s. Brains went from one pound to three pounds. The human brain became the most powerful in the world under conditions where motion was a constant evolutionary stimulus. Our brain grew under the influence of physical activity.

Are the learning abilities of someone in good physical condition different from those of someone in poor physical condition? And especially, will learning ability improve as physical conditioning improves? Many studies have been done, and there are great examples out there showing that when you're a couch potato, you will not age as well physically or mentally. That exercise helps brain function is based in our evolutionary history. Certainly exercise improves cardiovascular fitness, which in turn reduces the risk of diseases like heart attacks, strokes, obesity, and cancer.

A lifetime of exercise can result in a spontaneous, astonishing elevation in learning performance compared with those who are sedentary. Exercisers outperform couch potatoes in tests that measure long-term memory, reasoning, attention, problem solving, working, and both fluid and executive intelligence. Short-term memory does not appear to respond as well to physical activity as other types of memory. Certainly the degree of improvement varies from person to person.

The amount of exercise we're talking about is not that much. Brisk walking for thirty minutes a day is probably enough. You don't have to be a marathon runner. The body seems to be clamoring to go back to its evolutionary history millions of years ago. In the laboratory, the gold standard appears to be aerobics, thirty minutes at a clip, three to six times a week. Exercise is good for the brain.

In my experience as a neurosurgeon, a thirty-to-sixty minute brisk walk can be as good as taking a Prozac. Exercise can help anxiety, anger, and depression. The neurotransmitters serotonin, dopamine, and norepinephrine appear to be involved. Many psychiatrists now have begun adding a regimen of physical activity to the normal course of therapy.

On my website, **www.kachmannmindbody.com**, I have Rudy and Kelly's twenty prescriptions for stress reduction—exercise is one of them.

Scientific studies have shown that fluid intelligence, the type that involves problem-solving skills, was particularly hurt by a sedentary lifestyle.

Exercise improves children as well as adults. Physically fit children identified visual stimuli much faster than sedentary ones; it has also been proven among the elderly that exercises involving the senses—hearing, seeing, and balance—are greatly improved by exercise. Eating too many calories mostly produces free radicals, those nasty electrons that damage your brain cells and DNA. Exercise helps reduce those free radicals by increasing your blood flow and bringing more oxygen to your cells, eliminating the free radicals. Getting toxic electrons out obviously is a matter of access, which is why you need increased blood supply. The brain represents only about 2 percent of most people's body weight, and it accounts for about 20 percent of the body's total energy usage. Your brain needs a lot of glucose and generates a lot of toxic waste, which also means it needs a lot of oxygen-soaked blood, which you get from exercise. When you exercise, you increase blood flow across the tissues of your body. Exercise stimulates the blood vessels to create a powerful, flow-regulating molecule called nitric oxide. It enlarges your blood vessels and relaxes them, increasing your oxygen supply. The more you exercise, the more tissues you can feed, and the more tissues you can feed, the more toxic waste you can remove. This happens all over the body. Exercise improves the performance of most human functions.

Another brain-specific effect of exercise recently has become clear. At the molecular level, exercise also stimulates one of the brain's most powerful growth factors, BDNF (brain-derived neurotrophic factor), which aids in the development of healthy brain tissue. It increases the number of neurons and neurotransmitters. It produces neural genesis, new brain cells in the brain.

Physical exercise is like the fountain of youth and revitalizes your brain and body. The other day while getting a cup of coffee, a very nice fellow started talking to me. He was about my age, and he asked me when I was going to retire. I answered by saying, "The day after I die. I'm too busy to do that."

The benefits of exercise are system wide. It affects the main targets for vascular disease and diabetes, obesity, etc. It makes the muscles and bones stronger and improves our balance and strength. We're less likely to have a fall, which is a common cause of a lifetime in the nursing home. Exercise regulates your appetite, changes your blood lipid profile, and reduces the risk for cancer and autoimmune diseases. Exercise has a lot to do with your mental health. School systems of late are eliminating exercise programs, which is a major mistake, as it has been proven that exercise helps cognitive abilities. Exercise should be integrated into the school system and the workplace; it would improve performance and eliminate a lot illnesses and diseases.

Let's face it, our evolutionary history tells us: Our brains were built for walking. Improve your brainpower by exercising. Exercise gets blood to your brain, bringing it glucose to provide energy and oxygen to soak up the toxic electrons that are left over. It reduces oxidative stress and improves the function of our neurotransmitters. Exercising twice a week reduces your risk of general dementia by 60 percent.

How Much Exercise?

A HARVARD UNIVERSITY STUDY OF its graduate students indicated that a diet consisting of approximately two thousand calories combined with exercise has longevity and mental benefits. It really does matter. When you do aerobic exercise, you burn about three hundred calories a day.

That means walking briskly for about forty minutes would do the job. Walking slowly would take about seventy minutes, and pedaling on a stationary bike about thirty minutes. Exercise beyond that, some studies show, doesn't have that many health benefits.

As you can see, a small amount of exercise, for most individuals a brisk walk for little more than a half hour per day, will more than meet their requirements. Not surprisingly, this simple form of exercise also generates nearly a 70 percent reduction in the incidence of breast cancer in women.

You can see that moderate exercise is an exceptionally useful drug. It lowers excess blood glucose, and it lowers excess insulin since exercise requires the use of stored energy. Most of the stored energy will come from fat.

If some exercise is good, isn't a lot better? A more careful inspection of the longevity curve and exercise indicates that after about two thousand calories per week, the curve simply flattens out. As you increase exercise intensity, you also increase the levels of oxidative stress on the body. Remember those nasty free radicals, the result of oxidative stress on the body? Exercise requires a lot of oxygen, the big producer of free radicals. You're making more free radicals because your muscles require more ATP, which has its origins in food, the biggest producer of free radicals yet. Although you will be fitter, you probably won't live longer because of the excessive exercise (although Jack LaLanne will probably argue with you about that). The second reason is that the more intense the exercise, the greater the production of cortisol in response to that stress. So higher exercise intensity actually can increase two pillars of aging—free radicals and cortisone. If your goal is longevity, moderate exercise is your best course of action. The more intense the exercise, the faster the oxidative candle burns, and the more free radicals you produce.

Your function later in life will, of course, improve if you exercise regularly. You will have stronger muscles and bones and are less likely to take a fall and injure yourself. New functionality and quality of life in later years will strongly depend on exercise to preserve muscular strength.

The anti-aging benefits of exercise are mediated through two different hormone systems. The first hormonal system directly affects one of our four posts of aging, excess insulin. The reduction of insulin will be achieved primarily by aerobic exercise. Aerobic exercise simply means exercising at the intensity at which sufficient oxygen is delivered to the muscle to do the required work. As you age, your aerobic capacity decreases, which means you have to lower your intensity of exercise to maintain sufficient oxygen transfer to the muscles. The longer you exercise aerobically, the more you lower the insulin level.

Exercise builds muscle mass and is done by a growth hormone called testosterone. The secretion of these hormones will be increased by anaerobic exercise, exercise that is not as vigorous as aerobic exercise. Anaerobic exercise is any exercise whose intensity causes insufficient oxygen transfer to the muscle cells. This rapidly produces lactic acid as a breakdown product of glucose, which causes a burning sensation in the muscles.

Normally in aerobic exercise, muscles take blood glucose for their increased energy needs. Actively exercising muscles takes up nearly 30 percent more glucose than resting them. This uptake of blood glucose is a non-insulin-driving event. If there is not enough glucose or glycogen available during exercise, such as in a marathon run, then cortisone or stress predominates. The more effective the glucagon system is working to maintain blood glucose level, the less the backup systems are called into play. That is why lower-intensity aerobic exercise ensures that adequate blood glucose levels are maintained for the brain, thereby keeping the backup hormonal systems of adrenaline, and especially cortisol, in reserve. The more intense the exercise, the more growth hormone and testosterone are released. This occurs about fifteen to thirty minutes after the exercise has been completed. That is why anaerobic training, light weight lifting, and wind sprints are ideally suited for maximizing new muscle mass development. You must feel the burn in the muscles to achieve this. Growth hormone release is primarily needed to repair the micro tears in the muscles that occur during intense anaerobic exercise. Unfortunately, the more insulin in the bloodstream, the less growth hormone would be released, regardless of the intensity of your anaerobic training. That means that all the hormonal benefits of anaerobic exercise can quickly be undone by a high carbohydrate sports energy drink consumed just after exercise.

Exercise is important, but still not as important as eating the right diet. Your diet can impart a far greater effect on your anti-aging program than exercise alone. That is why you probably only need to exercise an hour per day, but remember, you can eat twenty-four hours per day. As a consequence, all the hormonal benefits of exercise may be offset by your diet. Dr. Barry Sears likes the 80/20 rule. Eighty percent of your benefits will come from diet; only 20 percent will come from exercise. Using the two together, you have a formal drug combination to lower insulin levels.

MATTHEW 7:13-14

"Enter by the narrow gate. For the gate is wide and the way is easy that leads to destruction, and those who enter by it are many. For the gate is narrow and the way is hard that leads to life, and those who find it are few.

Exercise and Diabetes

AS DR. FRANKLIN HOUSE SAYS, "Physical activity is medicine." It is well known throughout scientific medicine that weight loss, insulin resistance, and blood sugar levels are greatly affected by physical activity.

Of course, a plant-based diet (PBD) is equally important. You can exercise all you want, but it's doubtful that that alone will do the trick unless you're running marathons every week or swimming four hours a day.

Dr. Franklin House recommends strolling, stretching, strength and intermittent training.

I also recommend building muscle mass and strength because it has a great effect on your basic metabolic rate, BMR, increasing your resting caloric burn. The resting muscle uses about fifty to eighty calories a day per pound of muscle, a nice weight-loss benefit. Most of your sugar is metabolized in muscle and about 20 percent in the brain, and that greatly improves insulin resistance and lowers blood sugar.

Strolling after meals helps control blood sugar and combats insulin resistance. Stretching increases our flexibility. Strength training improves our metabolism and strengthens our bones. Intermittent training increases our endurance and gets us aerobically fit.

Even modest weight loss, five to 10 percent, can result in better glycemic control. A good physical program can even result in less need for insulin in type 1 diabetes.

Dr. House feels an increase in activity to be the cornerstone of diabetic care, as important as the diet. Remember, Dr. House has about thirty years of experience in the field in his clinic in Oklahoma.

That physical activity affects blood sugar control goes back to ancient times. The activity can slow pre-diabetes and even prevent type 2 diabetes. Physical activity, along with the plant-based diet, should be the foundation of diabetic treatment and prevention. Some medication may be necessary, but the aim should be to get rid of it.

Exercise causes glucose to be used for energy, mainly at the muscular level, the best place. Physical activity results in improved insulin sensitivity. Regular activity works in the long term through a process called improved glucose tolerance. The more active you are, the better you train your body to deal with sugar. The key to this process is glycogen, the storage form of glucose in the liver and muscle.

Physical activity slows insulin secretion from the pancreas, which causes the liver and muscles to use their stored glycogen to maintain the balance of glucose in the blood.

After physical activity, the glycogen stores in the liver and muscles have to be replenished, which means more glucose from the blood would be absorbed by the busy cells. This replacement can go on for twenty-four to forty-eight hours, until the glycogen is fully restored. Insulin sensitivity improves, and insulin pushes more glucose into the cells. Your blood sugar drops, and your type 2 diabetes is going away.

Physical activity combined with a high-nutrient diet is considered the most effective way to lose weight without having to restrict caloric intake or follow a starvation diet. With weight loss comes increase in insulin sensitivity, which allows you to reduce oral medication as well as insulin from shots. Insulin is a fat-growth hormone, and the less you have in your blood, the better.

Regular exercise also reduces heart attacks, strokes, cancer, dementia, and autoimmune disease. Physical activity also improves your brain function. Physical activity is important to the brain and the body and improves memory. You increase the blood supply to your brain, stimulate neural cell growth factors, and reduce inflammatory factors produced by fat, which cause dementia.

Exercise also reduces stress, so steroid levels, which are a great cause of obesity, drop. Stressed-out people have large bellies because steroids cause overeating and obesity. Exercise reduces depression and anxiety. A good walk is as good as taking a Prozac.

Of course, you should get clearance from your physician before you go on to a specific exercise program. Check your blood sugar frequently before, sometimes during, and after exercise, and sometimes much later, if you're not feeling well—especially if you switch to a plant-based diet. You have to be careful. If you change to a plant-based diet, I recommend giving it a couple weeks before going into a big-time exercise program because your blood sugar will be changing rapidly. For example, that's how Dr. House stops the oral medications on the first day in his plant-based eating program at his clinic. The blood sugars may drop quickly because you are getting rid of your disease. So the combination of exercise and eating properly can cause rapid changes in blood sugar, and you have to be careful.

In the person with lack of blood sugar control, less than 70 and greater than 250 can possibly lead to ketosis, which can lead to problems with the kidneys and liver and occasionally even cause loss of consciousness and death.

I recommend getting off the sad, mad toxic American diet first, then starting warm-ups, stretching, strolling, checking your blood sugar, starting lower-level weight training, and then going to aerobic activity slowly. Slowly increase activity over a month or two. If you have type 2 diabetes, you will see great benefits with a combination of proper eating and increased physical activity.

Certainly dyspnea, or shortness of breath, could mean you're overdoing it. So cut back a bit. Sometimes talk to your doctor. As a matter of fact, at the beginning of this program, be sure to get a clearance from a doctor and let him or her know what you're doing.

Avoid exercising at the peak of insulin action. Take your insulin one hour before physical activity. Watch for symptoms of low blood sugar during activity, feelings of shakiness, nervousness, and sweating. Check blood sugar every thirty minutes during activity, especially if it's a new activity. Stop if the blood sugar is less than seventy or if it's below seventy and you feel shaky, nervous, clammy, or confused. Take two glucose tablets or two pieces of hard candy, or drink four fluid ounces of fruit juice. Don't overdo it. Test again in fifteen minutes if you still have symptoms. You should watch for hypoglycemia for up to fifteen hours after your activity.

The Exercise Routine

- Five minutes of warm-up.
- Five minutes of stretching.
- A few minutes of strolling.
- Five minutes of weight lifting.
- Thirty to sixty minutes of aerobic activity.

Do this at least three times a week.

Exercise, Diabetes and History

Diabetes was first described by the Ebers Papyrus, written in 1500 BC by a German Egyptologist. Hippocrates, a Greek physician, also mentioned excessive urine flow. He also emphasized diet, exercise, and lifestyle. Around 1000 AD, a Greek physician prescribed exercise on horseback as a way to manage diabetes.

In 1857 Claude Bernard linked diabetes with glycogen metabolism. In 1889 Joseph Mehring and Oscar Mankowski found that dogs developed diabetes after the pancreas was removed.

Frederick Banting, from the University of Toronto, discovered insulin in 1923. Insulin does not cure diabetes so that people can live longer. Fifty years ago type 1 diabetes was the most common form of diabetes. Because of the mad toxic American diet, type 2 is now 90 percent of the diabetes problem, strictly related to being overweight and obese.

Diabetes mellitus is a group of diseases that affects metabolism, resulting from a defect in insulin production, either too little or too much. Glucose in the nervous system is the sole energy source, and also for working muscle groups, and is the primary fuel for exercise and physical activity. Insulin is a hormone secreted by the beta cells of the pancreas.

The rate of type 2 diabetes has increased 40 percent between 1997 and 2002. At this rate, it will double every ten years. Obesity has been the main problem.

Exercise needs to be a great priority. Only 39 percent of people with type 2 diabetes exercise on a regular basis, and we need to change that. Compare that with 58 percent of the nondiabetics who exercise regularly. The American College of Sports Medicine, ACSM, suggests that exercise is critical to reduce the progression of diabetic complications—strokes, heart attacks, amputations, blindness, renal disease. The ACSM suggests that exercise is effective in glucose control because it enhances the uptake of glucose. Exercising reduces the need for pills and shots for diabetes.

Lifestyle interventions seem to be at least as effective as drug therapy in preventing or delaying the progress of complications of diabetes. Lifestyle changes, including diet, can also prevent heart disease, strokes, dementia, cancer, and autoimmune diseases.

What happens during exercise? Several metabolic, hormonal, and cardiovascular changes occur during exercise. The carbohydrates you eat get stored in the liver and in muscles as glycogen. What you eat also contains fat, which gets stored as triglycerides in fat tissue. During exercise, you move your leg and arm muscles. Your heart is pumping at a faster rate, but a rush in blood flow increases to the active muscles. These muscles utilize stored energy without the use of oxygen. As you continue to exercise, oxygen supply becomes available to break down the carbohydrates, fat, and protein that can be used as energy for the continuous exercise. After possibly five to ten minutes, the liver becomes the main energy source for the active muscles and produces glucose. Glycogen stores in the muscles are depleted. After about twenty to thirty minutes of continuous exercise, free fatty acids, stored as triglycerides in fat tissue, are utilized in addition to the breakdown of glucose by the liver. Your muscles contract with exercise. Exercise causes the activation of glucose transport by GLUT 4. The protein carrier GLUT 4 helps increase glucose uptake by the active muscles.

Your body also secretes epinephrine, a growth hormone, as you exercise. Insulin secretion is reduced to facilitate production of glucose by the liver. Glucagon is also released to increase glucose production by the liver and glucose in the blood stream. At a moderate intensity of exercise, your body will utilize about 50 percent of the energy needed from carbohydrates. At a very high intensity of exercise, most of the energy used by your muscles will come from carbohydrates. As you finish your exercise session, your muscles will recover by continuously utilizing glucose twenty to forty hours after the exercise session is completed. That's important for diabetics to remember because you may become hypoglycemic many hours later.

Health Benefits of Exercise for People at Risk of Developing or Who Have Diabetes
- Improves glycemic control
- Increases metabolism and promotes weight loss
- Reduces risk of metabolic syndrome
- Improves insulin sensitivity

- Improves blood pressure
- Reduces diseases such as heart disease, strokes, cancer, and autoimmune disease
- Reduces stress and depression
- Increases muscular strength and muscle size
- Improves flexibility
- Improves aerobic capacity-VO2 max
- Reduces the need for a diabetes medication
- Increases bone density
- Avoids progression of peripheral neuropathy
- Reduces incidence of blindness, amputations, and renal transplants
- Reduces health care costs

Symptoms of Hyperglycemia

- Increased thirst
- Increased hunger
- Increased fatigue, weakness, malaise
- Increased urination
- Blurred vision
- Deep, rapid breathing
- Headache
- Nausea, vomiting, and abdominal pain
- No symptoms

Symptoms of Hypoglycemia

- Shaking, trembling
- Sweating
- Hunger, nausea

- Weakness
- Headache, dizziness
- Confusion, slow thinking, slurred speech, trouble concentrating
- Fatigue, sleepiness
- Blurred vision
- Fast pulse, pounding heart
- Tingling in extremities
- Heavy breathing
- No coordination
- No symptoms

Guidelines to be followed for people with diabetes

- Check your blood glucose before and after the exercise session. If you take insulin or certain diabetes pills, you are at risk for hypoglycemia during and after exercise and physical activity. If you're on insulin and your blood glucose before or after exercise is below 110, you should ingest 15-30 g of carbohydrate.
- If you're on diabetes pills, that puts you at risk for hypoglycemia, and if your blood glucose is below 90, you should ingest 50 to 30 g of carbohydrate.
- If you use daily injections, reduce the rapid-acting insulin dose by 30 to 50 percent by eating a meal closest to the exercise and physical activity to avoid hypoglycemia.
- If you are on an insulin pump, reduce your dose by 30 to 50 percent thirty to sixty minutes before exercise.
- If you have type 1 diabetes and your blood glucose before exercise is 250 mg or above, check for ketones.

- If your blood glucose level increases above the starting point value, be careful when taking a correcting dose.
- If you have type 2 diabetes and you're not feeling well, use insulin as described by your doctor. And if your blood glucose is close to four hundred, you should not exercise.
- Carry snacks that contain 15 to 30 g of carbohydrates, such as juice or glucose tablets, for the treatment of hypoglycemia.
- Drink fluids before, during, and after activity throughout the day.
- Avoid exercise in extreme heat.
- Avoid exercise in cold weather.
- Carry medical identification.
- If you take time off to heal, resume activity at a much lower intensity and progress slowly to a higher intensity.

Proper Stretching

A relaxed, sustained stretch with your attention focused on the muscles being stretched is very important. Don't bounce up and down.

- Stretch daily to increase joint mobility. Increasing joint mobility increases your range of motion.
- You should stretch all your muscle groups six days a week.
- Stretch your muscles when they're already warmed up.
- Spend more time on the stiff areas.
- Hold the stretch ten to thirty seconds. This is critical.
- Stretching should be static, not bouncy.
- Do it gently. If it hurts don't do it.
- Breathe deeply while you're stretching. It's relaxing.

Strength Training

- Warm up, take a brisk walk, or do another form of aerobic activity for five minutes.
- Test the maximal weight that you can lift at one time without hurting yourself and train at 50 to 80 percent of that; 80 percent will result in maximum improvement.
- Begin by doing one set of ten repetitions for each activity.
- As you progress, try two sets of ten, then three sets. When you're at three sets, increase the weight.
- Do this with as full a range of movement as possible.
- Remember that faster is not better.
- Use intermittent training, sixty seconds between sets. You'll find it's easier to do a hundred sit-ups if you do a set of ten, then rest for a ten count, then do another set, and so on, up to a count of one hundred.
- Begin workouts with the largest muscle groups and proceed to the smaller muscle structures—legs, back, and arms.
- Increases in muscle strength become easier when you do brief and infrequent training, so aim for strength training two to three times a week, not to exceed thirty minutes for each session.
- You must let you muscles recuperate after strength training. There should be at least forty-eight hours between workouts, but not more than ninety-six hours.
- Do strength training every other day. Stay focused.
- Correct breathing is important. Don't hold your breath when lifting weights.

Intermittent Training

Dr. Franklin House feels that intermittent training is the key to increasing physical activity among sedentary Americans. It is a non-continuous activity that incorporates an active rest for a fraction of a minute of moderate activity. Benefits from intermittent training come after only moderate intensity and short intervals of physical activity with rest. You make your body work a little, then you let it rest in little, then you make it work again, and so on. You do this by exerting five heartbeats above your target heart rate, then resting at five beats below your target heart rate. You don't stop the activity completely; you slow it down enough to rest. For example, you jog, then you walk—don't stop—and then you jog again. You might assume that during those rest periods, you'll be pretty much taking your time. I say again: you get the same health benefits if you rest during your activity as those who don't rest. Actually, you get added benefits—big ones—with intermittent training to get greater weight loss and greater body fat loss, too. This has been proven scientifically, and you're much more likely to participate in this way of training, as you don't have to have pain to gain.

Why It Works

Energy for activity comes from two basic metabolic sources: oxygen metabolism and anaerobic muscle metabolism. Anaerobic fitness is large bursts of energy in very short bits of time; sprinting or heavy lifting would qualify. The intensity of the activity exceeds the ability of the heart and lungs to get oxygen to the muscles being worked. So muscle metabolism is carried out anaerobically; anaerobic activity builds strength.

But what is the gold standard of health, fitness, and well-being? It's your VO2 Max that counts. That's where intermittent training comes in because practicing intermittent training, with its periods of rest after working at a high intensity, prevents the body from metabolizing anaerobically. Intermittent keeps the workout in the aerobic zone. That means any oxygen debt accumulated during the hard parts of the activity is paid back doing the rest intervals. Anaerobic activities are less painful and therefore easier to stick to for the long run.

Anaerobic activity uses glycogen, the form of sugar stored within muscle cells. Using glycogen produces `acid, or Lactaid, which in simple terms is the stuff that causes burning muscles during strenuous physical activity, decreases fat metabolism, and even contributes to a lack of motivation. When your workout is too intense, too hard, or too long, your body bypasses the aerobic phase in which it burns fat, and it burns glycogen instead, producing lactic acid. Again, intense physical exertion produces large amounts of lactic acid, especially in previously sedentary people. The more inactive you have been, the more it will hurt or burn your muscles if you suddenly start a vigorous activity. Those are great reasons to train intermittently.

Find your target heart rate and use it to train. Subtract your age in years from 220, then take that number and multiply it by .65. This is your target heart rate, Your training zone will be between five beats lower and five beats higher than your target heart rate. This is a simple method of determining your target heart rate and training zone.

Adjusting Your Training Intensity
- Set a goal to work out five or six days a week.

- Gradually increase the amount of time you're working out each day, up to sixty minutes a day.
- When you work for one hour, five or six days a week, gradually increase your training zone five beats per minute.
- You will eventually want to work up to 60 to 75 percent of your target heart rate.

Once you know your training zone, you can start your activity. Intermittent training is designed for use with cardiovascular activities such as walking, jogging, running, swimming, cross-country skiing, rolling, stair stepping, or even a walk thru Wal-Mart for a few minutes. Begin building up to your zone. If you get tired, slow down, then increase intensity again. You get the five beats permitted above your target heart rate.

ISAIAH 65:20

No more shall there be in it an infant who lives but a few days, or an old man who does not fill out his days, for the young man shall die a hundred years old, and the sinner a hundred years old shall be accursed.

Exercise and Rhythm

THE CONCEPT OF RHYTHM IS an integral part of life and is as old as history. Look at the old religions, tribal dancing, Hinduism. Dancing is thought to be the Arjun of the universe. In Hinduism, you've heard of the ancient cosmic dance of Shiva. The frequency and randomness of all such sounds are considered to hold healing powers, as is the vocalization "ohm." Apollo, the son of Zeus and the God of medicine, was known as a dancer. In Sparta, authorities require parents to instruct their children in the art of dancing, beginning at the age of five. Dancing is thought to be good for the body and overall health, as well as for the soul. In modern science, researchers have shown that music in rhythm produces measurable healing effects. Music has been proven to reduce stress and anxiety, as evidenced by moldable studies of heart patients who underwent catheterization and other unpleasant procedures. These patients' anxiety levels were significantly reduced when music was played during cardiac catheterization.

The brain uses rhythm to heal. It is important to breathe in rhythm because it affects our immunity. Healers across many different cultures have employed dance to induce a trance as part of a healing ritual. The Chinese discipline known as tai chi, which originated more than eight centuries ago, is still used as a healing art. Tai chi creates a meditative state that is set to restore natural rhythms and balance in the mind and the body. When you combine movement with rhythm, you enjoy the double benefit of exercise and the meditative state; you lower the inflammatory factors in the blood. It is better when you have a bit of low-back pain to do some rhythmic movement instead of lying in bed.

What action should you take?
- A 30 minute walk every day, in rhythm
- Swimming
- Entry-level aerobics and advance over time
- Ballroom dancing—I did it for two years with two Russian dancers.
- Biking
- Rowing
- Jogging
- Jumping rope
- Tap, hip-hop, square dancing
- Competitive sports
- Martial arts
- Get a personal trainer, when possible

PROVERBS 10:27
The fear of the Lord prolongs life, but the years of the wicked will be short.

Music and Longevity

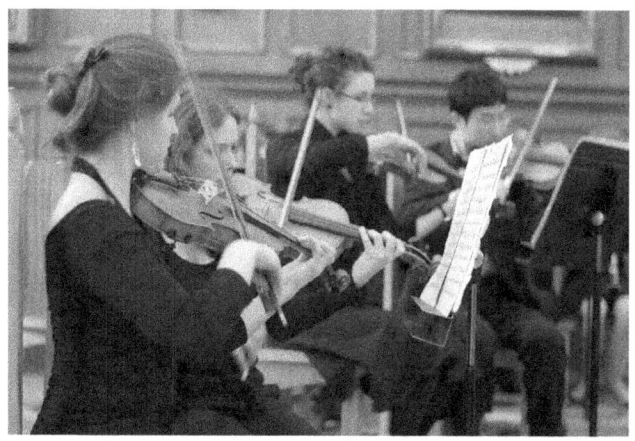

OUR INNER EARS ARE THE concert halls off our nervous system. The music fans out there are eager audiences of billions of neurons. Music can transform us to a higher level of brain integration. There is different music for different people.

Music can change mood quickly. Music lessons can improve our cognition; our ability to think improves. Dancing to music improves our longevity. Exercising to music causes brain cells to grow.

When I have my typical stressed-out day, I deal with life and death all day long: you have a malignant brain tumor; you're going to be paralyzed for life; how long do I have to live, Doctor? These are questions I face almost daily. These discussions have a great effect on me. Those problems are here today, and they will be here again tomorrow. How do I deal with that? How does the patient deal with that? As soon as I get in my car to drive across town to go to another hospital or play my friend in tennis, I turn on music that I enjoy, loud. I picked the music, and you know what? Within seconds, I am transformed. My neurons are firing a different tune, and maybe I'm singing to the music. I am visualizing the individual instruments being played; sometimes I'm conducting the orchestra. A friend of mine was driving behind me one time and called me on the phone. He said, "What are you doing waving those arms?" I said, "I'm conducting." One time I drove to the wrong town, listening to Pavarotti, when attending one of my neurosurgery clinics in Ohio. We all need these "pauses" in time. There's a reason they play music in the dental office.

It has been found that we learn better with music. The Mozart effect has been proven by scientific studies. Music makes us more intelligent. Our memory and learning ability improves with music, especially the music of Mozart. No one knows clearly why, and there is a lot of speculation as to the reason. Music and dancing can be traced in evolution. Even ancients danced and made music. Music is found in every culture. Extra pleasure and emotions can be found in music. Memories improve with emotions, and you're more likely to form long-term, explicit memories. Music improves our will to live.

I've provided the DVDs of Andre Rieu to a lot of nursing homes. I call them Rudy's concerts. Ten to fifteen people sit around in wheelchairs, watching the DVDs. Their happiness, alertness, and memories would improve for two or three days, according to the nurses. I always played them for my aging mother, and I know it lengthened her life and always put a smile on her face, and happiness leads to longevity. A Parkinson's disease patient may act almost normal as long as his favorite music is playing. Clearly this is a dopamine response.

Ecstasy is immediate pleasure. Music can do that. Music is the most immediate of all the arts and can produce ecstasy for a person in seconds. I experienced it once, when listening to Carmen singing "Mine Heisse Lippen from LeHare" with the Andre Rieu Orchestra.

Playing music—taking lessons—leads to stronger brain cells, increases our neurotransmitters, and gives us a longer life with a sound mind.

Sound affects the whole body. Music causes increased neurotransmitter activity in the nervous system, and the brain generates a flood of anticipation, which we use to make sense of melody, harmony, and rhythm. It takes us over. Music is beautiful; it imparts optimism in our soul and brings happiness. It heals us.

Music and art provide the mind with careful, ordered experience, not the chaos of a migraine. It's like a perfect sunrise. The world is too messy. Music brings coherence. Great beauty usually arises from greater complexity. We alter our view of the world, at least for a moment.

Nietzsche said this can be transcending. It puts us in another world for a moment, escaping our very chaotic inner world.

There are a number of ways that music affects us. It has been proven that music can slow down and equalize brain waves. Music affects our heartbeat, pulse rate, and blood pressure. It slows our stress response; we de-stress. Music reduces some muscle tension and improves body movement and coordination. That's why a lot of people exercise with music in their ears. For three or four minutes, play music while you do some stretching exercises. It will improve your movements and allow them to flow naturally. Lie down and listen to a slower movement or Mozart sympathy or a string quartet to relax you. Music can increase your endorphin levels, your own feel-good hormones. Music will strengthen your memory and learning.

When we are in our everyday activities, we use the beta waves of the brain. When relaxing, we are using our theta waves. When we are sleeping, we have delta a wave activity. Yoga, meditation, and music decrease the brainwave pattern and bring on theta wave activity, a more relaxing mode. We live longer if we control our stress. Playing music can balance our intellectual brain and increase productivity and creativity.

It has been proven that music can improve your immunity and help avoid cancer and infection. Fifty percent of mothers giving birth did not need anesthesia when listening to music. They studied the music of Mozart, Beethoven, the Beatles, and Bach, and Mozart was a winner in the learning process. They're not sure why, but it improved spatial perception, learning, and memory. Perhaps the rhythm, melody, and increased frequency of Mozart's music influenced the creative and learning regions of the brain. Mozart's music has creative and healing power. Mozart listened to his father's music while still in his mother's womb. Mozart said everything has been composed but not yet written down. What an imagination.

Bring music into your life. Listen, dance, sing, write, and promote it. Use CDs and DVDs and take dance and singing lessons. How powerful is your song? Mozart's music affects the electrical activity of the brain, according to the Royal Society of Medicine in London. It affects the hormones, the neurotransmitters and the neuropeptides, the communicators of the human brain.

PSALM 118:24

This is the day that the Lord has made; let us rejoice and be glad in it.

The Dance of Life

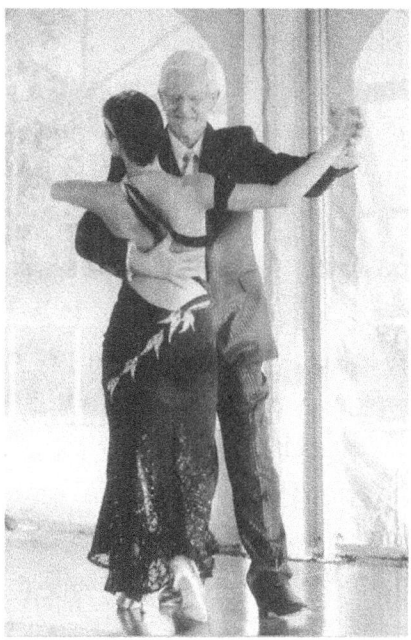

ALL TYPES OF DANCE ARE great. I'm speaking about the use of of rhythm and movement to improve your longevity and intelligence. You have to use your mind to dance correctly. Ballroom dancing improves the mind and the body. Join a class and do this one or two days a week regularly.

So whenever you are moving in rhythm, whether or not music is playing, you can consider yourself to be dancing. The dances of walking, jogging, biking, swimming, hiking, and even golf or tennis are following a rhythm. Keeping in rhythm means the timing of the swing, shot after shot, so you develop consistency. I play a lot of tennis. I have all my life, and really it's a form of dancing.

The effect of exercise on the immune system has been scientifically proven. Scientists have found that exercise has a direct effect on our white blood cells, the main cells affecting our immunity. After a few months of exercise, the levels of immunity-activating cytokines produced by white cells drop over 50 percent, while the levels of immunity-protecting cytokines rise about 35 percent, scientific studies have proven. Exercise is probably the single most effective way to lower inflammatory factors in the blood that cause cancer and vascular disease.

When physical activity is done through rhythm, it can be considered dance, a powerful way to get the most benefit from your exercise program. Pilates, for example, is an excellent way, as well as all other basic yoga activities. Chi-gong, tai chi, kundalini yoga, and dancing have the greatest effect on the inflammatory factors in your blood, the CRP (C-Reactive Protein) levels. Researchers have found greatly beneficial effects on anxiety and depression in people who performed exercises such as jogging, swimming, cycling, and walking. And music in rehabilitation and physical therapy programs for Parkinson's disease patients also have been shown to improve outcomes, when compared to standard physical exercises. Any rhythm to movement certainly increases the level of enjoyment and involvement in exercise classes. The addition of pumping rhythmic music to aerobic exercise classes encourages participation and increases satisfaction levels. Asked me and I will tell you—I own a yoga studio, and it works for our clients and us. Turning a standard exercise routine into a dance is more fun, less boring, and ensures that exercise is kept at their activity level.

Why does rhythmic exercise works so much better? RHYTHMIC contraction, alternating between flexion and extension, provides balance and strengthens both flexors and extensors equally. The nerve impulses that regulate muscle groups originate from signals in the brain and are transmitted along the spinal cord. With make movement rates of pattern in the brain and spinal cord that is also transmitted to our immune system. The same neurotransmitter chemicals released by a brain and nerve endings are sensed by our immune system. When a brain is dancing, so is our immune system. Human life itself consists of rhythms; it's quite possible that the immune system responds to these rhythms.

GALATIANS 1:4

Who gave himself for our sins to deliver us from the present evil age, according to the will of our God and Father,

Memory (The Nerve Cell—the Neuron)

WHAT IS THE MACHINERY OF memory? What makes it happen? Where is memory located? What is memory? The brain, which is largely made of essential fatty acids, is filled with signaling devices of a rather remarkable kind. There are wires and fuse boxes everywhere, one hundred billion neurons, one hundred trillion connecting devices. These signaling capabilities underlie all aspects of our memory, from recording sensations from the outside world to controlling movement, from the production of thought to the appreciation of a feeling. How do the neurons do that? We're really talking about the biological basis of behavior.

At the beginning of the twentieth century, the experimental work of Dr. Santiago Ramon Y Cajal, the great Spanish anatomist, formulated the "neuron doctrine," which states that the brain is made of discrete cells called nerve cells, or neurons, each with an external memory. He proposed that these neurons are the elementary signal units of the brain. He won the Nobel Prize in physiology or medicine for that in 1906.

The doctor pointed out that in all animals, there are three major types of nerve cells. Sensory neurons receive sensory information from the outside world for touch, vision, hearing, smell and taste. Motor neurons produce movement in various classes of interneurons and coordinate and integrate the flow of information in circuits. This was like the discovery of the computer and the Internet. Different numbers of neural cells were present in different living things. The snail might have twenty thousand neurons in the brain. The greater the complexity of the animal, the larger the number of neurons. A fruit fly has about three hundred thousand; a snail may have two thousand. A human has about one hundred billion.

Each neuron in the brain, in turn, makes about a thousand connections to other neurons at specialized connecting junctions called synapses. This means that any human brain has about one hundred trillion synaptic connections. One of the hallmarks of the modern biology of memory is the finding that the individual connection made between two neurons is an elementary unit of memory storage. I think we could say that we are our neurotransmitters; our selves are our neurotransmitters. The sum of a hundred trillion connections in the human brain provides one rough indicator of our maximal memory storage capacity.

The nature of the information conveyed by a nerve signal is determined not by the nature of the signal but by the particular pathway that the signal travels in the brain. We see the face of the person rather than hear his or her voice because the nerve cells in the retinas of our eyes connect to those parts of the brain, the visual system, that process and interpret visual information, informing us about what we see.

Dr. Cajal discovered that every neuron has four components: a cell body, a number of dendrites, an axon, and a family of axon terminations called the presynaptic terminals. The cell body is a large, globular central portion containing the nucleus, which in turn houses the DNA that encodes the neuron's genes. Surrounding the nucleus is the cytoplasm, which contains a variety of molecular machinery for sizing and packaging proteins necessary for the cell to function. The cell body gives rise to two types of long slender threads, or extensions, genetically known as nerve cell processes.

The Dendrites
and the Axon

THE DENDRITES TYPICALLY CONSIST OF elaborately branching processes that extend from the cell body, often in the form of a tree, and form the input component or receptive area for incoming signals. The axon, the output component of the neuron, is usually a singular process that extends from the cell body, and through neurotransmitters sends the information to the dendrites of the next cell.

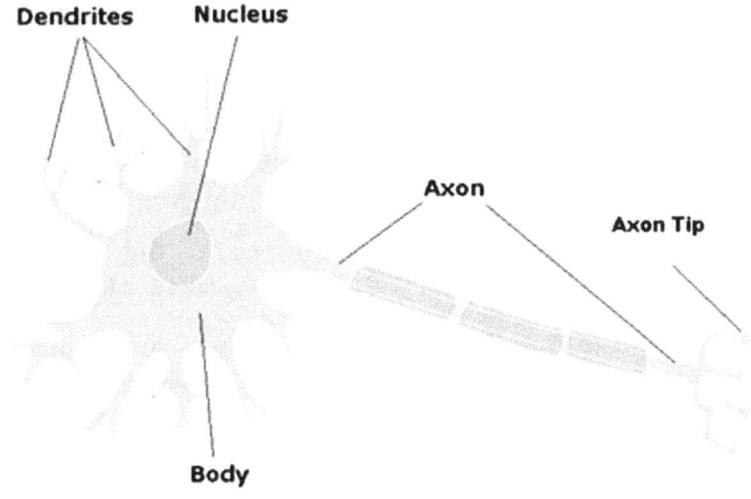

Depending on the cell-specific function, the axon can travel distances as short as .1 mm to as long as a meter or more from the spinal cord to the muscles of the toe. This anatomy was eventually clearly proven with the electron microscope. Neurons are dynamically polarized so that information flows in a predictable and consistent direction within each nerve cell through small electrical signals. Neurons have action potentials, which can be recorded within them, that are propagated by sodium, calcium, and potassium. These promote synaptic potentials that pass information from one nerve cell to another through the process of synaptic transmission. So information is passed along through action potentials and the chemicals of neurotransmitters.

The external plasma membrane of the cell maintains an arrest and electrical difference of about sixty-five millivolts. This is the resting potential. It results from an unequal distribution of sodium, potassium, and other chemicals across the cell membrane, so that the cell member membrane is negatively charged in the inside and positively on the outside. Action potentials and synaptic potentials result from changes in the membrane that cause the membrane potential to increase or decrease with respect to the resting membrane potential. The action potential is a change in the electrical potential across the external membrane of the cell created by the movement of sodium ions into the cell and the subsequent movement of potassium out of the cell through special pores in the cell membrane. The current produced by the action potential cannot jump directly across the synaptic cleft to activate the next dendrites. That is done by neurotransmitters output as the action potential reaches the presynaptic terminal. This signal leads to the release of a simple chemical substance. The neurotransmitter spills into the synaptic cleft or what acts as a signal through the dendrites of the next cell.

But where are our memories located? They are located in little vesicles—tiny packages, about five thousand molecules per vesicle—that are neurotransmitters. It is these molecules in these vesicles that are our memory.

These small vesicles, which carry our neurotransmitters, carry a single quantum of synaptic transmitter—as already stated about five thousand—and they are released to stimulate the dendrites of the next cell. It was a Sir Bernard Katz, a British neurophysicist, who pioneered the modern analysis of synaptic transmission. He discovered that chemical synaptic transmitters are released not as single molecules, but by multi-molecular packets containing about five thousand molecules. Each packet is called a quantum and is contained in a cellular organelle called the synaptic vesicle. This is well demonstrated on an electron microscope.

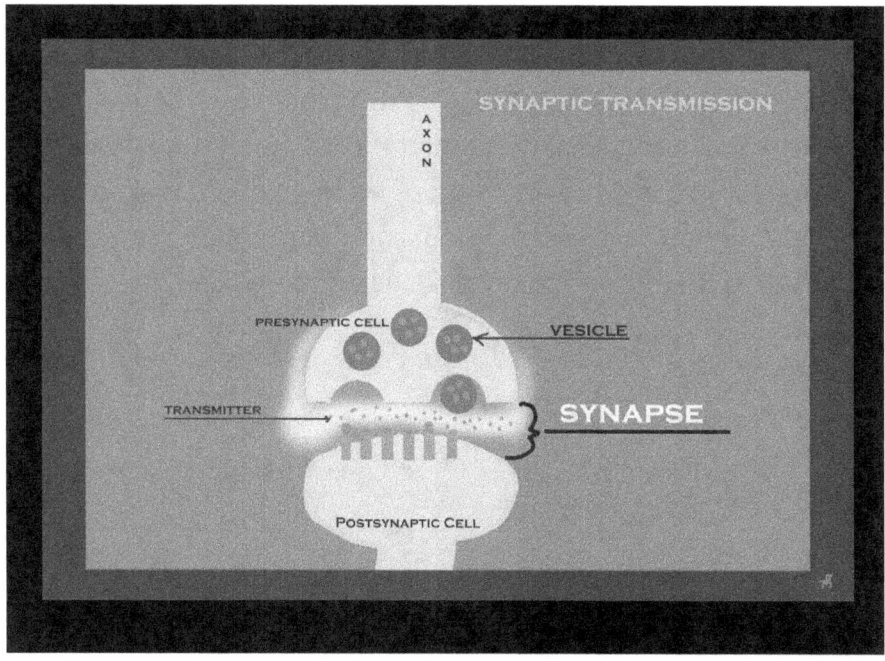

Once released into the synaptic cleft, the five thousand molecules of chemical transmitter diffuse to the postsynaptic target cell to protein molecules called receptors, which are located on the cell surface. Each class of neurotransmitter molecules is capable of being mechanized by a number of different receptors. Dr. Cajal predicted that the learning process might alter the patterns and intensities of signals that constitute the brain's activity. As a result of this altered activity, neurons should be able to modulate the ability to communicate with one another. The process of these alterations in basic synaptic communication was then called synaptic plasticity. Now we speak a lot about neural plasticity—that we can improve our learning and memory by using it, diet, and many other ways, as found in my Longevity Body-Memory Index.

It was Dr. Sherrington who actually coined the term synapse, which comes from the Greek word meaning to fast or to embrace. Dr. Sherrington had the great insight to appreciate that aplastic change at synapses, along the lines suggested by Dr. Cajal, could be responsible for the habituation he observed in the limb-withdrawal reflex. A lot of these studies were done in marine snails, which contained only twenty thousand neural cells, compared to mice, which had three hundred thousand nerve cells.

ROMANS 13:11

Besides this you know the time, that the hour has come for you to wake from sleep. For salvation is nearer to us now than when we first believed.

What Is Memory?

WHAT IS MEMORY? IT IS using our five senses to gather information, then storing it, and then retrieving it.

Our brain is our most important physical possession. And our memory is our being and identity. It is our intelligence, personality, and humanity. Not fulfilling your brain's potential is a tragedy.

This is the age of the brain. It has been proven that the brain can grow and increase its synapses. Even in old age, we can grow a few thousand brain cells each day. Contrary to previous popular opinion, in old age we can have a tremendous increase in our neurotransmitters. By using our brain in education, reading, activity, exercise, and the latest computer technology, we can do brain aerobics and improve the function of our brain. It's called neural plasticity.

The brain is our primary resource, and our intelligence is our currency.

Life in the information age is based on memory and intellect. We must stimulate the brain to its full capacity. Just as we exercise the body, we must exercise our brain. We need to be in "cognitive brain change."

Memory is about brain cells and neurotransmitters. Our identity is the neuron and neurotransmitters. Our intellect is determined by our brain cells and neurotransmitters. We have over one hundred billion neural cells and one hundred trillion synapses; every neuron is filled with DNA, our genetic messenger. We have many dendrites, the receiving branches, like a tree, of the next neural cell and a single axon for every cell. The dendrites have receptors, at least one thousand, that receive the incoming signals from the previous axon. The axon carries little quantum packages of molecules, about five thousand per vesicle, to the synaptic site. That's where your memory is located. The end of the axon has terminals with these tiny vesicles full of neurotransmitters that send a message to the next cell's dendrites across the synaptic cleft. That's where the transport center is located, the fuse box. The more synapses, the more information processing.

Each neuron has myriad synapses, and they communicate with hundreds of thousands of other neurons in milliseconds. By increasing our connections, we are improving our memory. The more neurons and neurotransmitters you have, the greater your memory power.

What are we made of? Who are we? What is the self? What is our own self-identity? What makes our ego? It's our memories of our family and us. Without memories we are blank pages. I remember my ninety-three-year-old mother struggling to figure out who we were, and even perhaps who she was, at a Christmas party. She had very little to say, observing the scene, and I alone wondered, what did she really comprehend? Was it cognitive mental impairment? Dementia? Advanced dementia? We never used those terms on her, and she lived to age ninety-seven without any of us ever using those nasty terms of memory loss or whatever it was. We just loved her and took care of her and thought it was part of getting a day older, and we were glad she was around. She never said or did anything unusual. She just smiled at us and appreciated everything we did for her. I always brought a lot of music, and that perked her up. From my experience I never thought the medications for dementia worked very well. I never gave them to her. That was even before I read the excellent book by Dr. Peter Whitehouse. She had a good life and died at age ninety-seven when her heart just stopped. We are but a memory as time goes by.

What is normal aging? What type of memory systems do we really have? Is it normal to lose 50 percent of our memory by age eighty-five, as it is often said?

What good is it to live to be a hundred if you're not of sound mind? is a common question. I hear that a lot. My belief is that our brainpower, the majority of the time, is determined by what we do with it—our choices.

What type of memory systems do we have? Life without memory is no life at all, some would say. I'm not sure about that. Memory is our reason, our feeling, even our action. Transience is the inability to hold onto information. About 90 percent of what we hear or read we don't remember very long, and that is normal.

We have short-term memories and long-term memories. They are stored in different parts of the brain, and parts of it are commonly shared. Short-term memories are stored in the hippo-campus; emotional memories are stored in the amygdale; long-term memories are stored all over the brain.

The ability to learn and remember are the hallmarks of mem-ory. We need an intact brain to fully function because many parts of the brain are involved with this task. We know that short-term memory is mostly stored in the hippocampus because Dr. Sco-ville removed the hippocampus on the right and left side in a patient called H. M. for epilepsy. That patient completely lost his short-term memory. But he still retained the implicit long-term memory. Long-term memory is divided into implicit and explicit memory. Playing a game of tennis, for example—something fairly automatic based on past training—is called implicit or non-declarative memory. Explicit memory or declarative memory is like remembering a college reunion.

A brain consists of neurons, nerve cells, support cells, and chemical neurotransmitters with electric impulses in which our memories are encoded in molecules, stored, and retrieved as a result of neurotransmitter and chemical interactions. We have one hundred billion brain cells and one hundred trillion synaptic neurotransmitter interactions.

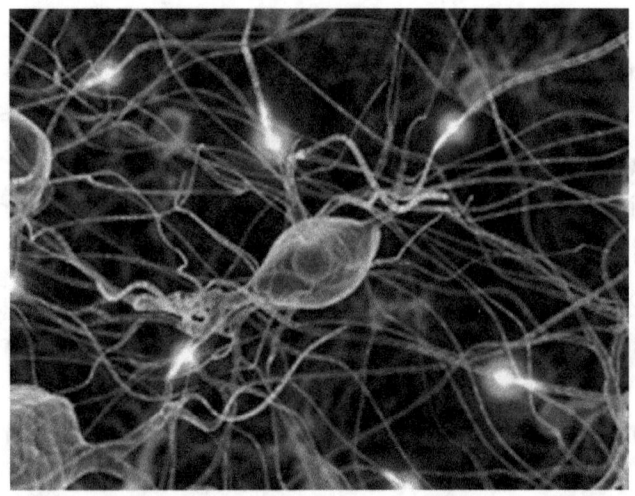

We have trillions of synaptic connections, and each neuron has about two hundred thousand synapses. Examples of neurotransmitters are serotonin, dopamine, and GABA. We store information on a molecular level. We think and remember with our neurotransmitters. They can be altered with brain activity. See Rudy's Longevity Body-Mind Index (LBMI).

We first receive information, which is processed in short-term memory. That is the switching station or control center. We usually lose most immediate memory quickly, but this is not stored unless we pay special attention to it and encode it. Only a small percentage of information makes it to long-term memory. You have to organize and rehearse it to get it to long-term memory. It helps to know memory skills. Information is better remembered if we use all our senses of hearing, vision, touch, etc. Visualization helps encode memory for the long term. Once information is stored in long-term memory, it may become permanent. Short-term memory has only limited capacity. Long-term memory is bigger.

Recall is retrieving long-term memory. Patients with short-term memory loss may have recall for long-term memory. You see that especially in the elderly, and even in advanced dementia (AD).

The immediate memory is short-term memory. Working memory is activities that we carry out every day. Short-term memory is converted to long-term memory at the molecular level.

The brain's hippocampus is located in the medial temporal lobe; it's shaped like a seahorse. We have a hippocampus on each side of the brain. It is extremely important in memory.

When the brain converts immediate memory into permanent memory, it's like wiring in a computer hard drive. The hippocampus interacts with the cerebral cortex.

Emotional situations affect memory more than auditory or visual cues. Emotional memories of information are easier to learn and retrieve.

Memory with Age

RECALLING NAMES, DATES, THE LOCATION of keys and household objects, recent and past events, meetings, and appointments, becomes more difficult as we get older.

Age-related memory loss is more commonly associated with recent events than past ones. It almost amazes me that my mother could recite poetry from high school all day long. Before the age of television, they must've spent a lot of time on poetry. I always felt she could recite a whole book, but ask her what month it was, and she probably could not tell you.

Age slows down learning ability and recall skills. It is more difficult to learn math and music. We drive more slowly. Talking on the phone, texting, and driving are certainly not compatible with aging, no less with teenagers. Two days ago I was almost run over by a teenager texting and driving into McDonald's, where I was getting a cup of coffee. Multitasking gets more difficult. Mental aerobics can help. Age-associated memory loss can be checked with a simple test. It's about 40 percent by age fifty, 50 percent by age sixty, and about 70 percent by age seventy and older. No one knows the exact rate. Memory loss is generally divided into aged-associated memory loss, cognitive memory loss, and dementia. All of these, of course, increase with age. Language skills at twenty may predict Alzheimer's disease at seventy. Intelligent and educated people have less dementia. As we age, synapses don't work as well, and miscommunications may occur.

A brain may shrink about 10 percent by age sixty-five. But head injuries, such as from accidents and football or soccer, can lead to memory loss and dementia.

Our aging brain accumulates amyloidal plaques and neuro-fibrillary tangles. It is thought these collections occur from cell death and brain degeneration. A few neurophysiologists think this process could possibly be repaired. They have been demonstrated at biopsies and autopsies. They have been demonstrated on functional MRIs and PET scans and SPEC scans. There are no clear-cut pathological findings for Alzheimer's disease. It is a diagnosis of exclusion, not 100 percent certain with minimal cognitive impairment. You see amyloidal and neurofibrillary tangles, but in less concentration. They start in the temporal lobe and spread to the parietal. Alzheimer's disease doubles every five years in the sixty-five-to-ninety-year range. By 110, maybe I'll have it—I don't believe it. Is this normal aging? Women's brains are smaller than men's, but they have more important gray matter. Let's face it: they are smarter than we.

Memory is the ability to recall what happened to us a day ago, a week ago, or years ago. Long-term declarative memory is a story. The information asked for is explicitly available for recollection. Remembering a play or a song, or a sports game, or a poem like my mother repeated all day, is implicit memory. She demonstrated it beautifully. I bet she knew a hundred poems completely accurately. But I could not be sure she could remember my name. She had great implicit and non-declarative memory. That's certainly speaks well for my tennis game. It's funny: I was playing my friend Dr. John Crawford, my main tennis competitor, yesterday. He's younger and slightly better than I. The whole match, I was trying to get him into declarative memory from non-declarative memory. In other words, I wanted him to not play thoughtlessly and start thinking instead, and sure enough, in the second set he started talking to himself, and things got worse for him. Very interesting. Your explicit long-term memory may be poor, but you can still play your favorite sport, or repeat your favorite poem, or play the piano regularly.

ACTS 17:30-31

The times of ignorance God overlooked, but now he commands all people everywhere to repent, because he has fixed a day on which he will judge the world in righteousness by a man whom he has appointed; and of this he has given assurance to all by raising him from the dead."

Improving Your Memory

WHAT'S SOMETHING YOU COULD DO quickly to improve your memory skills? Something you could use immediately? We all need help with this. Remembering a name has always been difficult for me, because I pay no attention to it in the first place. I'm a very busy person. I realize that's no excuse. I've been working with the system designed by Dr. Gary Small, director of the UCLA Center of aging.

Coding of memory is a way of filing the information in a place so you can retrieve it later. Our memories are more effective if we attach some emotion or importance to the information or just do it in a methodical manner as taught by Dr. Gary Small. Also, we have to listen to the information in the first place. How could you possibly remember the name if you didn't hear it the first time? The information has to have some meaning to you. My problem has been that what I do has life and death attached to it. Remember I'm an actively practicing neurosurgeon. I did four operations yesterday and I was 74 on Sunday. Because so much information is coming to me on a daily basis, I don't think I really hear things said to me or encode them in my brain, unless something very important is attached to that piece of information. I love my patients, when usually they have fairly serious problems, so meeting someone else doesn't have that much meaning to me. And I probably don't really hear the name in the first place. I probably barely looked at the person and didn't connect.

Twenty years ago, the unusual case of the paralyzed man in the emergency room, or the child that was dying from a shunt and I drilled a hole in the head to save his life on the spot, I remembered decades later, like it happened today. I also say "never forget some else's complications". I never do because I put importance to it. I'm learning something without it being my patient. But your name, I may not know it every time, but, I will remember the meaning you have in my life

Sad, but true. But I'm learning and changing. Dr. Gary Small's book has done that for me.

Meaning is hardwired in our brain. Emotions are hardwired in our brain. The greater the emotional attachment, the greater the meaning. And if you heard the information in the first place, you are much more likely to remember it.

Dr. Small would say "look," "snap," and "connect." Really have a good look at who you are talking to, and actually listened to what they have to say. Our powerful five senses and our sixth sense, emotion, is a powerful first step. Then actively look and visualize something distinctive about that person, their hair, their nose, their clothes, etc. Visualization is the language of the unconscious mind and trying to visualize the memory is very important. The great memory experts use visualization all the time. Let it become a habit. Visualization is a great memory technique.

The true art of memory is paying attention in the first place. This is very important, just as driving home is. That's what I don't do in the first place, but I'm getting better at it. Mentally stay in the driver's seat.

"Looking" is the second basic skill after listening and paying attention. A sense of listening, visualization, sense of smell and touch is a good start in trying to remember something. Use all your senses. Snap great mental snapshots of your memories. As you visualize the image, you are already developing the second basic skill—snap. You are creating a mental snapshot of information you wish to remember. Afterwards, you just pull out the snapshot and describe what you see. Creating vivid and memorable images fixes them into our long-term memory storage. Snaps can take two forms, real or imagined. Our brain does not know the difference. Imagined snaps can be fantasy, distortion, an image you observe.

Recently, while on vacation in Naples Florida I was looking for a tennis match. The secretary at the club and hotel said no pro was available, but there was a guest who was willing to play. He came out and said my name is Philippe De Monte Bello. Turns out he was the CEO of the Metropolitan Museum of Art for 30 years. A name I certainly did not want to forget, so I looked, snapped and connected, the Dr. Gary Small way. Certainly, it was not hard to do since I attached a lot of emotion and importance to this individual. He gave a lecture that night at the hotel and it was great. What a nice person and a fascinating individual. You can see I'm putting my lesson to work. Of course also, I've repeated the story many times to my friends. That, of course, impressed it further in my long-term memory. Repetition is very important for long-term memory.

Developing techniques to connect mental snaps together is a basic element of nearly all memory techniques. Connect is the process of associating to mental snaps and you can remember that connection later. This will help you to remember birthdates, the names of employees' spouses, and allow you never again to forget the name connected to the face. To connect to snaps, simply create a brand-new snap that connects both mental images. Place one image on top of the other, and make one image rotate or dance around the other. Have one image crash or penetrate the other. Merge images together, wrap one image around the other. Connect is the basis of the link method, which orders items by associating the things to be remembered with each other. The ideas and images become part of a chain, starting with the first item. Linking them is often hard, when we need to remember lists of unrelated things to do, particularly if writing out that list is inconvenient or impossible. That's how a waiter at a restaurant does that and then quickly forgets the information. He just needs to remember it to the kitchen. The most effective links of associations are the ones we create ourselves, particularly those stemming from a first association. Another application of connect is the use of acronyms or the creation of words for the first letters of items to be remembered.

Practice using "look", "snap" and "connect" and your basic everyday memory skills will improve. Look—actively observe what you want to learn. Slow down, take notice, and focus on what you want to remember. Snap—great mental snapshots of memories. To read a mental snapshot of the visual information you wish to remember. Connect—link mental snapshots together and associate the images to be remembered in a chain, starting with the first image, which is associated with the second.

Stress and Longevity

IS STRESS GOOD OR BAD for you? Clearly, acute stress can save your life; you avoid the oncoming truck. But it can also kill you; you suffer a heart attack after you lose your job. Chronic stress is making Americans sick, causing a lot of illness and leading to shorter lives.

Chronic, long-term stress can give you mind-body diseases (see mind-body index) and give you a lot of bad health. Overeating, lack of exercise, and sleepless nights can lead to bad habits such as smoking, alcohol, and drugs. So stress can shorten your life and seriously affect the condition of your brain. Alcohol and drugs can shrink your brain; they destroy neurons and neurotransmitters.

Stress can destroy your immune system, and you develop infections much more commonly, including all inflammatory diseases and autoimmune diseases. Arthritis, multiple sclerosis, cancers, and viral and bacterial illnesses are much more common in stressed individuals. You're much more likely to have a cold when you're living under constant stress. Cancer or heart attack is sometimes the answer to the death of a spouse.

When I started in neurosurgery and had no partners, I worked day and night. Usually on Saturdays in the afternoon, I would start running a temperature. This occurred every week, and it was over after little bit of rest on Sundays. When my first partner came, it went away. Guess what? He had never worked so hard, and he developed the same problem. When our third partner arrived, the second partner's Saturday temperature went away— a good example of stress.

It's how we think that counts. Our thoughts affect our sixty trillion body cells. It is our neurotransmitters, hormones, and neuropeptides. Our sixty trillion body cells also affect our brain. Brain-body, body-brain. We can destroy ourselves with our thought processes, leading to chronic illness and death.

The cortisone in our body produced by stress can bring eicosanoid production to a screeching halt. The eicosanoids are the Intel chips of our body, the super hormones that regulate the physiology in an organized and coherent manner. The chemical cortisone produced by stress inhibits the chemical phospholipase 1; phospholipase 1 is the enzyme responsible for the release of all the essential fatty acid from the cell. That is how stress through cortisone destroys our body.

When you look at the cultures around the world where people live a lot longer, you can see that they have a lot less stress. The family dinner at a definite time, the outdoor café for a glass of wine, walking, exercise, lots of music, love of the family, a strong faith—that all leads to less stressful living and longer lives.

About 90 percent of all American adults experience high stress levels at least one to two times a week. One in four Americans have crushing stress every day. A survey of Americans would reveal that 57 percent feel excessive stress much or most of the time.

The best definition of stress is "the inability to cope with threats (real or imaginary) to our physical, social, emotional, and spiritual well-being." In the end our immune and nervous systems are affected most by stress. Our health is dependent on how we think. We can control how we react. Let me give you an example. Two Arabs are racing in their huge Mercedes in the desert had a huge head-on collision. They both survived and jumped out of their cars. Instead of beating up on each other verbally or physically, they profusely hugged each other. They said if the accident had not occurred, they never would have met. This is a good story to remember.

I bring it up as a story many times in my life. How you perceive stress is how stress affects you. The key to good health is learning how to turn bad stress into good stress. Stress occurs when there is change and we are forced to adapt to that change. Change occurs constantly, and stress just "is." So stress can make us ill and even kill us. It can destroy our body. We need to learn how to handle it. Distress affects almost all body systems, resulting in cardiovascular and neuromuscular disorders and many mind-body illnesses.

There Are Seventeen Phases to the Stress Response

1. The cerebral cortex receives a message.
2. It sends a message to the hypothalamus.
3. The hypothalamus cortisone releases the hormone CRH.
4. CRH stimulates the pituitary gland.
5. The pituitary gland releases ACTH.
6. ACTH stimulates the adrenal gland.
7. The adrenal gland releases cortisol, adrenalin, and other chemicals.
8. The thyroid gland releases hormones.
9. Sex hormones are reduced.
10. The digestive tract shuts down.
11. Sugar is released into the bloodstream.
12. Cholesterol is released into the bloodstream from the liver.
13. The heart begins racing, and blood pressure goes up.
14. The breathing rate increases.
15. The blood thickens and coagulates more readily.
16. The skin blanches and sweats.
17. The five senses become more acute, and the pupils dilate.

It is the accumulation of stress stored in our subconscious mind that causes mind-body illnesses as well as a general stress response.

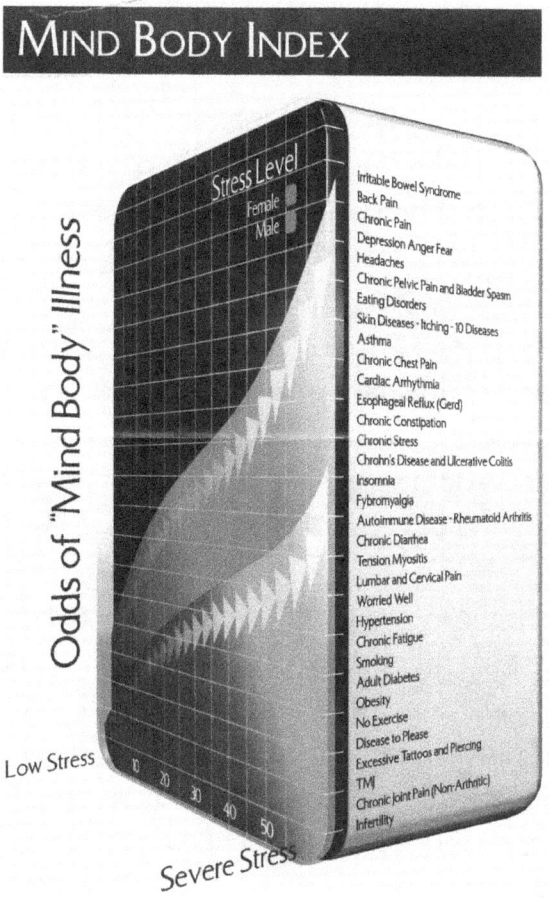

*Significant changes in life patterns of an individual will develop the most stress. You can see the stress test events that caused the most stress. Yes, we can even predict who has the highest chance of developing a mind-body illnesses using the **Mind-Body Index** above.*

It has been found that stress can even cause cancer. Dr. Lawrence La Shan, a psychiatrist who treated advanced cancer patients for forty-five years, wrote a very nice book on that. The doctor viewed fifty patients who had been hospitalized for cancer. La Shan was fascinated by the striking similarity in the life history of the cancer patients. He also found that he could double the life span of most of his patients with advanced cancer if he could give them the will to live and get them to practice stress-reduction techniques. His practice was three blocks from my home as a child in New York. I never met him, but I have one very interesting story. He would take an advanced breast cancer patient to lunch once a month at the Metropolitan Museum of Art, which was just down the street from me. They would walk for one half hour through the Museum of Art after lunch, looking at her favorite art. After five years of doing this, he studied her and found no evidence of cancer in her body. I wish I had met Dr. La Shan.

Changes occur in the hippocampus as a result of excessive cortisol that mimic the result of aging. As we grow older, we are less able to regulate our stress response, and as a result, levels of cortisol, as produced during stress, don't return to normal for longer periods of time. Under these conditions, the aged can suffer rapid destruction of brain cells. Stress can actually play a role in the development and progression of Alzheimer's disease. Stress can also interfere with our fertility when we're younger or our sex life when we are older. The most serious result of chronic high cortisone levels is the suppression of the immune system. High stress levels can cause shrinkage of the spleen and thymus. They are vital for the production of white cells and our immunity.

Dr. Hans Selye in Canada did the original studies on chronic stress. That resulted in his famous adaptation syndrome. When studying rats, he found that placing them under stress affected their blood pressure, heart, thymus gland, adrenal gland, and white blood cells, eventually leading to death.

We need to have a program to fight stress every day if we expect to live a long, mentally strong life. From making a plan—exercise, music, love of the family, meditation, yoga exercises—and facing up to the problems that we have in a realistic manner, there is always an answer. When you find it, your stress will be reduced, no matter how bad the situation is.

People who've had the most severe stress in their lives and survived it, such as concentration camp victims, developed a sense of commitment, control, hardiness, and a sense of coherence as to what was happening to them. See my website: *www.kachmannmindbody.com* for my twenty prescriptions to reduce stress.

1. CREATE A SPIRITUAL, SAFE PLACE IN THE HOME.
a. Do three minutes of abdominal breathing that is calm and focused.

2. MEDITATE.
a. Concentrate on your nasal breath.
b. Next, concentrate on your abdomen going up and down.
c. Say or chant a mantra (mind energy) multiple times. For example: Spirit, God, Om, Sat Nam, Let Go, Be Free, I'm Happy, etc.

3. VISUALIZE AN IMAGE DAILY OF WHAT YOU WANT TO ACHIEVE THAT DAY OR IN THE FUTURE.

4. SAY SOMETHING THANKFUL WHEN YOU GO TO BED EVERY NIGHT, AND SAY SOMETHING OPTIMISTIC OR JOYFUL EVERY MORNING.

5. MANAGE YOUR FINANCES WELL BECAUSE IT IS ONE OF THE BIGGEST CAUSES OF STRESS.

a. Get your finances organized.

b. Don't panic and remember to breathe.

c. Be disciplined and know your debts.

d. Make a new plan by thinking your way out of it and seeing a new way of making it.

6. DON'T FOCUS ON NEGATIVITY.

a. Avoid TV, radio, and bad news media. Media fast.

b. Don't spend the whole night on the computer or watching TV. Give yourself time to transition into sleep—read a book, relax, let the mind unwind.

c. News/media are preoccupied with gloom and doom, crime, world pain, murder, mayhem and perversion. Give it a rest.

7. PRACTICE YOGA, TAI CHI, WALKING, OR DANCING, OR ENJOY EXERCISES THAT BRING ABOUT RELAXATION AND MEDITATION RATHER THAN OVERSTRESSING THE BODY AND MIND.

8. EACH DAY, SPEND FIFTEEN TO THIRTY MINUTES PRACTICING MEDITATIVE WALKING—"WALKING MEDITATION."

a. Use your senses to explore the present moment.

b. Appreciate sounds, appreciate what you see, and appreciate nature.

9. THINK POSITIVELY.
a. Be hard-headed and tough-minded; refuse to let others bring you down.
b. Don't give up; believe in yourself.
c. Make a plan to solve the problem.
d. Write a plan and visualize it daily.

10. LIVE IN THE PRESENT MOMENT, NOT IN THE FUTURE OR PAST
a. Live in the light of the day, not in the storm of yesterday and tsunami of tomorrow.

11. ENJOY MUSIC IN YOUR HOME AND IN YOUR CAR ON THE WAY TO WORK AND BACK.
a. It is the language of God or Spirit.
b. Music sound is medicine. It is the bridge between spirit and matter.

12. EAT PROPER FOOD.
a. Food is a drug. Don't abuse it.
b. Don't use food to manage your psychology because it is not a good stress reducer.
c. Read *The Secret of the Non-Diet*. It is about proper food selection.

13. ORGANIZE YOUR TIME.
a. Demand at least fifteen to thirty minutes for yourself daily, no matter what the situation is.

14. TREAT YOURSELF TO A MASSAGE. LET GO OF THE MONKEY MIND

a. Take a mind shampoo and clean your mind of stress daily. How you think is everything.

15. DON'T SMOKE, USE ILLEGAL DRUGS, OR TAKE EXCESSIVE MEDICATIONS.
a. In the long run, they will cause stress.

16. FALL IN LOVE WITH YOURSELF AND APPRECIATE THE LOVE OF THE FAMILY NO MATTER WHAT THE PROBLEMS ARE.

17. BE A HAPPY PERSON.
a. Avoid negative thoughts or statements. No one can solve all the world's problems, so don't focus on them.

18. LIVE A LIFE OF GRATITUDE RATHER THAN A LIFE OF REGRET.
a. You can't change the past.
b. Say nice things to people all day such as "You look great," "Have a nice day," or "Thank you again."

19. LET GO OF SELF-JUDGMENT AND SELF-CRITICISM.
a. You are the creation of spirit or God. He does not make mistakes.

20. KNOW WHAT MIND-BODY ILLNESSES OR STRESS RELATED ILLNESSES ARE.
a. Stress causes 75 percent of the illnesses that we see doctors about. Wellness and stress education is what you need 75 percent of the time.
b. Avoid unnecessary tests and procedures.
c. By understanding what the illnesses are, I have gathered them together in the Mind-Body Index.

d. Read *Welcome to your Mind Body*. It will save you money in medical care, reduce your stress, and cure your problems with the proper techniques as recommended above.

ACTS 3:19
Repent therefore, and turn again, that your sins may be blotted out,

The Neurobiology of Stress

Future shock [is] the shattering stress and disorientation that we Induce in individuals by subjecting them to too much change in too short a time.

– Alvin Toffler

LESS THAN A CENTURY AGO, the word "stress" wasn't a part of the American lexicon. Engineers working on the Brooklyn Bridge in Lower Manhattan understood the technical term as "mechanical forces acting on physical structures." According to linguist, author, and pundit William Safire, stress, the noun, is a shortening of distress, rooted in the Latin *distringere*, "to hinder, molest." Stress, the verb, has another root as well: the Latin *stringere*, "to draw tight, press together," which is related to strain. Today stress has come to take its meaning from the verb pressure: either through direct force, tension exerted on a person or thing." Pressure, tension, and stress, which are synonymous in general use, lead to anxiety and strain. The vogue term was presaged by John Locke circa 1698: "Though the faculties of the mind are improved by exercise, yet they must not be put to a stress beyond their strength."

Stress is the inability to cope with a *perceived* (real or imagined) threat to one's mental, physical, emotional, and spiritual well-being, which results in a series of physiological responses and adaptations. Internal stressors can also be physical (infections, inflammation) or psychological. External stressors include adverse physical conditions (such as pain or hot or cold temperatures) or stressful psychological environments. Medically speaking, stress is the nonspecific response of the body to any demand. The presence of stress causes measurable physical changes such as increases in pulse, respiration, and heart rate. Virtually all systems—cardiovascular, pulmonary, digestive, endocrine, immune, and nervous—act to meet the perceived danger. Stress has replaced infectious agents of disease as the number-one health evil facing Western culture.

In the 1920s, physiologist Walter Cannon first used the term "stress" to describe the body's response to unpleasant conditions, named the fight-or-flight response. Cannon described in his classic *The Wisdom of the Body* that the body had automatic control over functions such as temperature control, digestion, and heart rate. A single nerve, called the vagus, which exits at the back of the brain and continues down the body via the spinal cord and nerve branches, can send signals to the body's organs, including the pupils of the eyes, the salivary glands, the heart, the bronchi of the lungs, the stomach, the intestines, the bladder, the sex organs and the adrenal glands. When Cannon stimulated the vagus nerve through electrodes implanted in the brain's hypothalamus just above the pituitary gland, he discovered that there were physiological changes in all of these organs consistent with the body's response to an emergency. Blood, for example, was rerouted from the internal organs of digestion to the muscles. An increase of adrenaline stimulated the heart and caused the liver to release extra sugar for instant energy.

Acute stress stimulates the sympathetic adrenal system and an outpouring of adrenalin-like hormones that prepare the body for fight or flight. Pupils dilate, blood pressure and heart rate rise, and blood flow to the brain increases, resulting in improved vision and other cerebral functions. Glycogen stores in the liver rapidly break down into glucose to provide immediate energy. Blood shunts from the gut to the muscles of the arms and legs so that we can run faster. Blood also clots more rapidly to diminish loss from any hemorrhage. In short, a host of potentially life-saving physiological and chemical events occur under the body's stress response.

Hans Selye, a charismatic and influential neuroendocrinologist, popularized the notion that stress (and the emotional or physical reaction to it) can make people sick. Building on Cannon's model of the fight-or-flight response to a generalized notion of stress, Selye proposed that over time, harsh environments (including the stress of modern living) can cause increasing levels of physical stress, eventually resulting in physical syndromes, exhaustion, and even death. In his landmark study published in 1950, *The Physiology and Pathology of Exposure to Stress*, Selye theorized that poor adaptation to stress was the basis of most illnesses and disease. His theories permeated medical thinking and influenced medical research for twenty years, replacing psychoanalytically based psychosomatic theories.

About ten years later, physicist Elmer Green developed biofeedback techniques in which patients learned to control unconscious processes. Under his care, patients watched monitoring devices that tracked things like heart rate or blood pressure. By observing how their different actions affected data readouts, patients could start to voluntarily regulate certain body functions such as blood pressure. Green's experience led him to state:

Every change in the physiological state is accompanied by an appropriate change in the mental emotional state, conscious or unconscious, and conversely, every change in the emotional state, conscious or unconscious, is accompanied by an appropriate change in the physiological state.

Herbert Benson found that under most circumstances, once the acute threat has passed, the response becomes inactivated, and levels of stress hormones return to normal, a condition called the relaxation response. The problem is that contemporary life poses ongoing stressful situations that are not short lived, and the urge to act (to fight or to flee) must be suppressed or the fight-or-flight response becomes perpetual.

The physiology of stress and the fight-or-flight response has been studied and publicized more than any other neurochemical process. The body's stress response activates the brain's hypothalamus and pituitary glands, which regulate hormones, particularly the stress hormone cortisol that regulates immune functioning, blood pressure, insulin, and proper glucose metabolism. While small increases in cortisol improve performance, long-term (chronic) exposure to stress hormones can cause atrophy of the brain's hippocampus, leading to memory impairment. To make matters worse, we pour adrenalin into our bodies with cans of popular energy drinks; doubleshot, threepump, and grande cafe lattes; or popular movies and television shows—all of which causes our body and mind to endure even more stress. High cortisol levels also increase food intake and contribute to central body fat, a condition my colleagues in cardiology refer to as "toxic fat." Abdominal fat, insulin resistance or glucose intolerance, high blood pressure, inflammation, and bad cholesterol are known to increase the progression of heart disease.

Prolonged stress also can be hazardous to brain function, hormone production, immune responses, and other processes. Stress-related disorders and diseases brought on or worsened by psychological stress commonly involve the autonomic nervous system, which controls the body's internal organs, including the heart, lungs, and brain.

Chronically stressed individuals have increased levels of the stress hormone cortisol, which slows the delivery of immune cells and molecules to injury sites. In turn, this slows the start of the healing process. In 2004, a twenty-year-long study proved that the longer the duration of a stressor, the greater the disruption of proinflammatory cytokines, which in turn may increase susceptibility to viruses that cause the common cold. The study also showed that social relationships may influence wellness and recovery from disease. Social isolation such as loneliness raised blood pressure. Alzheimer's caregivers were more likely to have severe colds. Bereavement and unemployment lowered lymphocyte counts up to two months after the initial stressor. Couples going through a divorce have depressed T and NK cells, immune cells that strengthen resistance to infection. And research on wound healing suggests that marital stress delays healing and increases the body's production of proinflammatory cytokines that can accelerate a range of age-related diseases such as heart disease. Depressing life events such as divorce or the death of a loved one can even create enough stress to interfere with the heart's pump, causing "broken heart syndrome," a temporary heart failure that can lead to death if not treated.

People are more susceptible to illness when under stress, including young students, who create fewer antibodies to the flu vaccine around exam time. When the reasons for patients' visits to physicians are examined, 60-90 percent of visits are related to stress and other psychosocial factors. In my own practice, I've discovered that a ten-minute "stress survey" is an important diagnostic tool. Physicians need to integrate stress evaluations into standard history taking and examinations.

America's advanced technical society is responsible for much of the information overload that causes stress, and generalized anxiety will affect all adults to some degree at different points in their lives. The constant influx of information from mass communication systems such as blogging, video teleconferencing, mobile phones, e-mail, snail mail, text messaging, instant messaging, landlines, advertisements, telemarketers, and voicemail, as well as the information output from the Internet, newspapers, magazines, newsletters, billboards, satellite television, and radio causes a certain degree of information angst in everyone. Consider life in America only a hundred years ago: Only 8 percent of homes had a telephone; eight thousand cars were on the road; the speed limit was 10 mph; and there were only 144 miles of paved roads. Today the information highway connects people across the planet, opening the door not just to our neighboring country's cultural nuances, but to the complex socioeconomic realities of second- and third-world countries that seemed remote—but the impact of 9/11 will forever remind us that the world is in our backyard. Our hearts and minds haven't caught up with technology's great lurch forward.

Stress levels rise for different reasons and in different seasons, around national holidays and periods of economic instability and recession. Post-9/11, a nationwide survey published in the *NEJM* found that 90 percent of American adults experienced a stress-related symptom. Following an economic recession, the Department of Health, Education, and the Infectious Disease Center in Atlanta revealed nationwide increases in ulcers, heart attacks, impotency, weight loss, and depression. You may want to consider heading to the tanning booth the next time you're feeling in a funk. Light therapy and even tanning booths have been shown to raise serotonin levels in the skin and can help people who suffer from seasonal affective disorder.

Job stress is one of the most universal and chronic kinds of stress. Technically, job stress is "lack of harmony between the individual and his or her work environment." Employment losses are often followed by an increase in heart attacks, hypertension, ulcers, and other pain-related illnesses—and even death. Factory work and jet lag are known to create discordance between natural body rhythms and daily activities, resulting in disordered sleep patterns, mood disorders, and other medical problems. In factory work, the risk of accidental injury is significantly increased during the night shift. Perhaps more disturbing is a recent report that destruction of the brain's master clock rendered mice more susceptible to experimentally induced cancers.

The American idolization of youth in media such as films and television programs and marketing or advertisements also creates a kind of unconscious stress. In contrast to many Eastern countries such as China and Japan, older Americans are unsupported by family members, who are often scattered all over the country or overwhelmed with their immediate responsibilities. Foreigners often criticize Americans for consigning the aged disabled to nursing homes or senior citizen communities, a concept that doesn't exist in most countries.

Time-pressured activity is another common cause of stress. The Earth moves on a twenty-four-hour cycle, and so do we. Our body clocks synchronize us to our environment, and even to the seasons' changing day lengths. For this we can thank circadian rhythms, temporal programs of around twenty-four hours found in virtually all living things. Their most obvious signature is our sleep-wake cycles. But research on a wide range of organisms is revealing many clocks, working at levels from the cellular to the whole animal.

The body's main circadian pacemaker is found deep within the brain's hypothalamus, which receives direct input from the retina. A recently discovered class of photoreceptors not involved in image generation contains a light-sensitive pigment. Even blind people lacking functional vision can respond to light signals with the retina's photoreceptors. The brain's "master clock" orchestrates a wide range of neural and hormonal signals that drive a multitude of cyclical responses around the body, making routine sleep a critical component of rejuvenation and wellness.

Adding to stress is the fact that organized religion has waned drastically in modern Western society, leaving people stranded in a materialistic society with no clear belief system. A general feeling of incompleteness or spiritual vacuum haunts many people today, promoting a degree of confusion in values. The popular spiritual debate between scientists and people of faith may make some people feel they have to choose sides: the cold, fact-filled universe of biological evolution or the supernatural world of miracles and faith. St. Augustine, one of the greatest Western thinkers, warns against a narrow perspective of the creation story in Genesis. In my opinion, the human spirit requires neither religion nor reliance on miracles;

the inherent quality or particularity to the human condition is the result of wondrous adaptive biological mechanisms that protect, sustain, and perpetuate our existence—although spirituality and beliefs are great producers of immunity and happiness.

Stress and
High Blood Pressure

HIGH BLOOD PRESSURE OFTEN OCCURS earlier in life, is more severe, and has more complications in African American men and women. And yet, blacks are less likely to seek treatment until their blood pressure has been high for so long that vital organs have already started to suffer damage. Denial is often a component in seeking treatment, but so are lack of access to medical care, misdiagnosis, lack of awareness about inexpensive preventative self-care, and dismissive doctors. Women, especially, have no feeling of empowerment when it comes to their own health care. And for good reason—several studies have shown that when it comes to women, physicians don't listen as well and don't prescribe preventative medications as much, diagnostic tests aren't as accurate, and women's symptoms are harder to recognize.

A terrible case example took place in 2006 when forty-nine-year-old Beatrice arrived at an emergency room in Ohio complaining of nausea, shortness of breath, and chest pains. A nurse saw her briefly and told her to wait. Her daughter twice told the hospital staff that her mother needed immediate care. But two hours later, when Beatrice's name was finally called, the staff found her slumped in a chair, already dead. Patients suffering from an apparent heart attack must be put on cardiac monitoring immediately, within ten minutes of their arrival. The coroner said in Beatrice's case, none of that happened. A coroner's jury investigating the case ruled Beatrice's death a homicide, opening the door for criminal prosecution.

Critical delays in the detection, accurate diagnosis, and proper treatment of vascular diseases threaten women's lives. The racial disparity in survival for disease and illness is multifactorial, and the more we learn about the origins, both genetic and environmental, the more capable doctors will be in developing more tailored screening and preventive and therapeutic strategies for high-risk patients in the future. The pioneering neurosurgeon Harvey Cushing said almost a century ago, "A physician must consider more than a diseased organ, more than the whole person; the physician must view the person in his or her world."

African Americans on average have *double* the rate of hypertension in comparison to whites. Among the reasons for such disparities, we might consider the stress experienced by African Americans striving to overcome negative stereotypes and prove themselves against a backdrop of racism and inequality, about which they are acutely aware. Our reactions to others have far-reaching biological impacts, triggering a cascade of destructive or positive internal chemicals. Under stress, the body shuts down resources from the endocrine and immune systems and releases hormones that fuel the body to act. These hormones also trigger inflammatory mechanisms known to influence the development of diabetes and hypertension. The elevation of inflammation is likely a key reason why metabolic syndrome leads to accelerated coronary disease risk in women.

Acute Manifestations
of Stress

EVERYONE HAS A STORY RELATED to stress. My most notable one is about Scott, then a globetrotting, Google-clicking, dot-com executive. Scott headed the nuts and bolts of developing an online service in China, which was not an easy feat when you consider Beijing's obsession to control free speech over an Internet spanning half a billion users. He had been flying back and forth to Asia to carve out the terms of a multimillion-dollar deal with China's largest PC manufacturer. Two weeks spent in the purple pollution haze of Beijing would send most people to the hospital, but Scott went about his business and rushed home in time for a wedding. Upon arriving stateside after the fourteen-hour flight, his back began to itch. When he took off his shirt and asked his wife to look at the rash with a copy of the consumer edition of *The Merck Manual* in hand, she diagnosed him with shingles. Shingles is caused by the varicellazoster virus, the same virus that causes chickenpox. After you've had chickenpox, the virus lies dormant in your nerves. Years later, the virus may reactivate under stress.

A week later, Scott woke up with a fever, stiff neck, and the worst headache of his life. His wife left a bridal shower to take him to the emergency room, where he was evaluated for meningitis, an infection and inflammation of the membranes (meninges) and cerebrospinal fluid surrounding your brain and spinal cord. Meningitis is a rare complication of shingles. When I arrived at the hospital, Scott laid in the dark on a gurney with a bucket beside his head. He was overcome by pain so severe that he vomited continuously, making a spinal tap to confirm the diagnosis "difficult." After testing positive for viral meningitis (bacterial meningitis can progress to widespread infection of the nervous system, leading to shock and death within days), I ordered an IV with the antiviral medication Val acyclovir and morphine. Complications of meningitis include permanent hearing loss, blindness, loss of speech, and brain damage, leading to paralysis or even death.

Shingles is rare for people under fifty years old. You're more susceptible to shingles if you have cancer or a weakened immune system. I asked Scott's wife, a thin woman with a tall forehead and large blue eyes, if he was under a lot of stress. She told me that day in and day out for months, Scott had bowed to business demands in more ways than one. He was making the fourteen-hour flight from Washington, DC, to Beijing so often that he earned the prestigious 1K status in mileage awards. His cell phone, computer, and Blackberry buzzed late in the evening and early in the morning because of the twelve-hour time difference in business hours. She said she could often hear Scott raising his voice and repeating himself on nightly conference calls in their library, irritated with translators who often botched key terms in English, resulting in confusion and delays.

After a week in the hospital and several weeks of in-home nursing care, Scott fully recovered. Because I was concerned that he may have brushed up against a rare disease from a region famous for breeding deadly pandemics, I referred him to an "international" epidemiologist for a battery of tests. His blood work was 100 percent normal, implying that his shingles had been triggered by stress.

As Scott's story illustrates, stress is your body's perception of a physical or psychological threat and being ill-prepared for it. The fight-or-flight response results in your body's release of stress hormones—adrenaline or noradrenalin. The short-term impact of stress includes increased metabolic, heart, and breathing rates. The long-term, chronic impact can be a weakened immune system, cardiac arrhythmias, hypertension, abdominal cramping and diarrhea, and muscle tension. Inflammatory diseases that are shown to be associated with an abrupt stress response are rheumatoid arthritis, Lupus, dermatitis, and asthma.

Healing Stress-Related Illness

LEARNED ATTITUDES THROUGH CULTURAL, RELIGIOUS, and family experiences strongly influence the way people adapt to stress. Everyone has a highly complex set of beliefs and attitudes. Each one of us sees things, including stress, in a totally different way.

Current pharmaceutical and surgical approaches cannot adequately treat stress-related illness. Holistic mind-body approaches, including nutrition, exercise, and the motivation of patients to change their belief structures, can help people better cope with the endemic stress of our culture. Most adults operate on a level of necessary and tolerable stress to improve performance. However, excessive, long-term stress reaction can lead to illness and disease or nonphysical pain syndromes. Our physiology wasn't created or didn't evolve fast enough to cope with the burden of the kind of repeated stress and anxiety prevalent today. Emotions affect which details we remember. And things that trigger strong emotional responses—like stressful car accidents or violent images on television—are recalled more readily, according to renowned psychologist Kevin Ochsner.

Ochsner's research at Columbia University examines the psychological and neural processes involved in extracting emotional and cognitive meaning from the world. His research interests include the psychological and neural processes involved in emotion, pain, and selfhood using neuroscience methods such as fMRI and the study of brain lesion populations. Perhaps one of the most valuable findings of his research is that when we're experiencing something disturbing, our brain records more details than if we were experiencing something relaxing or pleasurable.

Over a century ago, Freud proposed that people could exclude unwanted memories from awareness, a process called "repression." It was unknown, however, how repression occurred in the brain. Ochsner's team used fMRI to identify the neural systems involved in keeping unwanted memories out of awareness. Controlling unwanted memories was associated with increased prefrontal activation, reduced activation of the hippocampus, and impaired retention of those memories, confirming the existence of an active forgetting process and establishing a neurobiological model for guiding inquiry into motivated forgetting. This provides a psychological model for the voluntary form of repression (suppression) proposed by Freud.

One theory for stress-related illness is that it results from repression of stress or stress-related memories. That is, part of our brain wants to react while another part tries to restrain, which results in tension. The thinking part of your brain—the prefrontal lobes located in the front part of your brain—doesn't allow you to scream out. (Think of Edvard Munch's painting The Scream). The amygdala would have us screaming and jumping from tree to tree. A lot of your negative thoughts and emotions about stress are stored in the subconscious, the unconscious part of your mind where memories, feelings, or thoughts influence your behavior without your awareness. This is the key when dealing with stress-related illnesses. According to John Sarno, MD:

Your brain tries to shove any threatening emotions into your unconscious so you don't have to become aware of them. When the feelings aren't all that intense or threatening, your brain manages to keep them repressed. However, when the emotions are particularly strong, it's harder to keep them tucked away, so your brain needs to create a distraction. It creates real physiological changes in your body, which in turn creates real symptoms. These symptoms are painful or distressing enough to take your attention away from the threatening, unacceptable feelings.

Prolonged stress and the conditioned impulse to restrain negative emotions such as anger or frustration can produce incremental changes in the brain and immune system over many years. Emotional tension related to repression of negative memories, emotion, and stress contributes to the majority of pain-related, psychogenic illness—the symptoms become a distraction from the original stimulus.

Stress-provoking images, sounds, and situations can cause people (especially children) to overproduce stress hormones, including the adrenal hormone cortisol, which is responsible for much of the physical damage caused by long-term stress. Chronic elevations of stress hormones contribute to a host of illnesses, including asthma, gastric ulcers, and cardiovascular disease. Children who are shy or inhibited in unfamiliar situations have been shown to suffer from multiple allergic disorders. Some of the most disturbing research on stress is showing that persistent elevations of cortisol increases the vulnerability of neurons in the hippocampus to damage by other substances; this brain region influences motivation, memory, and emotion.

The body's stress response operates autonomously but can be conditioned through the techniques we discuss in Part IV. To better understand the mechanics of stress, you'll need to learn a few simple insights about the brain's multitasking functionality and the body's process of activating the stress response.

Mapping Stress

STRESS STARTS WITH A PERCEIVED threat, the root of all fear, which causes the body's fight-or-flight response. The adrenal glands send adrenalin, noradrenalin, and cortisol into the bloodstream, quickening the heartbeat and raising blood pressure. The sympathetic nervous system helps redirect blood to the muscles, constricting arteries and reducing blood flow to the internal organs. Fat cells are released into the bloodstream for quick energy, which are not all reabsorbed. The release of stress hormones makes blood platelets stickier, which might lead to the accumulation of plaque. This process occurs over and over in people who are easily stressed. But in the chronically angry, the damage is amplified because the response itself is sharper.

Using a "hostility questionnaire" and angiograms, researchers have found that most hostile men have more severe arteriosclerosis. Researchers at the University of Miami recently found that HIV-positive people who took part in stress management workshops showed improved endocrine and immune functions.

Specific brain and body regions process fear, emotions, and the physiological stress response. The brain is divided into the cerebrum, diencephalons, brain stem, and cerebellum. Three interconnected brain regions regulate fear: the prefrontal cortex, the amygdala, and the hypothalamus.

The frontal lobes of the cerebrum, including the prefrontal cortex, make up 60 percent of the brain hemispheres and extend from the back of the eyes to the middle of the ears. The prefrontal cortex interprets sensory stimuli and evaluates potential danger. The frontal lobes are the "executive planning center" of the brain, enabling us to calculate, coordinate, and plan. When trauma or disease affects the frontal lobes, we may become apathetic, lethargic, and unable to start or complete new tasks. Some of us may become uninhibited and start gambling impulsively and recklessly, becoming obsessed sexually and picking fights.

The second region involved in fear and aggression is the amygdala, almond shaped regions in the limbic system. Limbic means border. The limbic system borders the cortex (upper part of the brain) and the subcortex (lower part of the brain). The amygdala performs a primary role in the processing and memory of emotional reactions. Infants are born with well-developed amygdala, which is why a baby cries when picked up by an unfamiliar person or taken to an unfamiliar place. Fear is a primitive survival tactic. Autistics have a highly reduced amygdala; they are unable to process several emotions, including the comprehension of fear or aggression in people's faces or behavioral expressions. The stimulus-seeking behavior and lack of inhibition associated with Attention Deficit Hyperactivity Disorder also may be due to disrupted connections between the amygdala and frontal cortex. The amygdala is your key to intuition.

Neuroscientists think that the amygdala reacts without input from the thinking part of the brain. An emotional reaction like fear can more easily gain control over the cortex and influence cortical processes than the cortex can gain control over the amygdala. During a stressful event, the amygdala sends impulses to the hypothalamus for activation of the sympathetic nervous system and other important brain regions for increased reflexes, facial expressions, and activation of dopamine and adrenaline hormones.

Sometimes emotions can be triggered without the cortex knowing exactly what's going on. Neuroscientists refer to these emotional explosions as "neural hijackings." A key emotional area deep in the center of the brain, once again the amygdala, proclaims an emergency, recruiting the rest of the mind and body to act. The hijacking occurs in an instant, overriding the thinking or judging part of the brain, the neocortex. Today, one in twenty Americans may be susceptible to repeated, uncontrollable emotional outbursts in which they lash out with physical abuse, road rage, or other unjustifiably violent actions. Scientists at Harvard and the University of Chicago say that neural hijackings are on the rise, and substance abuse is a typically a complicating factor. In some people with mental disorders, this may be especially strong, so their emotions are being triggered in ways that prevent them from having insight into what they are doing.

Fear follows two simultaneous paths in the brain: 1) the *unconscious*, intuitive recognition of danger flashes in the amygdala, and 2) the *conscious* executive decision making that takes place in the prefrontal cortex. The amygdala also performs primary roles in the formation and storage of detailed memories associated with emotional events. Military members in the Middle East have to be alert for surprise attacks anyplace, anytime. The emotional and psychological conditioning can have lasting effects. For example, after the Afghan War, one of my friends said that the long, drooping clusters of Spanish moss on the live oak trees in his backyard became ominous; they were ideal perches with camouflage for snipers. He removed the long, grayish green filaments of moss. Studies on posttraumatic stress disorder connect an overabundance of fear memories in the amygdala with an inability to consciously discriminate danger from harmless phenomena.

The centrally located diencephalons in the brain include the thalamus, hypothalamus, and epithalamus. The thalamus is about 80 percent of the diencephalons and serves as a critical relay station for sensory impulses, except for the sense of smell. The thalamus receives visual information from the eyes, auditory information from the ears, and sensory information from the body. It processes and analyzes this information and then relays it for further processing. The hypothalamus is a small region below the thalamus.

The main function of the hypothalamus is homeostasis, or maintaining the body's status quo. Factors such as blood pressure, body temperature, fluid and electrolyte balance, and body weight are held to a precise value called the setpoint. Although this setpoint can migrate over time, from day to day it is remarkably fixed. Many doctors still believe the hypothalamus is the chief center governing the emotional aspect of human life. More current research supports the interaction of the brain's structures, neuropeptides, hormones, and neurotransmitters to create the chemical, electrical, and physiologic state of the living organism. There can be differences of opinion about this, but most neurologists and neurosurgeons, as well as the rest of the medical community, still do not appreciate the great influence of neuropeptides on the body.

A substantial portion of human cellular machinery is dedicated to maintaining homeostasis. In response to stress signals from the amygdala, the hypothalamus secretes corticotrophin-releasing hormone (CRH). This is a key hormone shared by the central nervous system and immune system, uniting the stress and immune responses. CRH triggers the pituitary gland to secrete adrenocorticotropic hormone (ACTH), which in turn spurs the adrenal gland to produce cortisol.

Cortisol is a steroid hormone that helps you meet the demands of stress. It's also a potent anti-inflammatory agent, playing a critical role in preventing the immune system from damaging tissues. Cortisol is essential, so its levels in the blood are closely controlled. When cortisol levels rise, ACTH levels normally fall. When cortisol levels fall, ACTH levels normally rise. The body's response to cortisol is to increase blood pressure and to decrease the pulse rate. Other internal changes include a decrease in the number of white blood cells and an increase in the rate that amino acids (protein) change into sugar (glucose). CRH and cortisol are two important keys to the mind-body connection.

CRH-secreting neurons of the hypothalamus regulate the autonomic nervous center (ANS), as well as the locus ceruleus, an area of the brain stem involved in arousal, fear, and enhanced vigilance. The ANS is an entire little brain unto itself; its name comes from "autonomous," and it runs bodily functions without our awareness or control, although we can consciously alter it through techniques such as focus, meditation, and breathing exercises. The ANS includes two systems that often oppose each other: the sympathetic and parasympathetic systems.

The parasympathetic system has many specific functions, including slowing the heart, constricting the pupils, stimulating the gut and salivary glands, and other responses that are not a priority when threatened by danger. The body's parasympathetic, or the relaxation response, can be solicited through soothing music, laughter, nature, and other inexpensive, non-pharmaceutical techniques such as breathing deeply. The sympathetic system evokes responses characteristic of the fight-or-flight response when pupils dilate, muscles tense, heart rate increases, and the digestive system is put on hold. It also stimulates immune organs, such as the spleen. Our knowledge about how the brain processes emotion has been gleaned through the study of the stress response. We'll give you the "play-by-play" of a familiar scene to provide a glimpse into your internal disaster response team.

You're driving and talking on your cell phone. The right parietal lobes of your brain help judge spatial relationships, and the frontal lobe provides judgment and decision making. Your conscience (somewhere in your neocortex) prevents you from driving like a maniac. Suddenly, the car in front of you swerves, and a two-hundred-pound buck appears standing in the middle of the road, antlers and all.

When confronting a frightening "no-eye-contact" situation, animals freeze, remaining completely still for prolonged periods. Inhibiting motion reduces the likelihood of attack (except in this case, the "attacker" is a two-ton SUV barreling down the highway at 60 mph).

At the sight of the deer, nerves from your retina transmit sensory data to the visual thalamus, then to the cortex and amygdala deep within the limbic system. Interactions in the cortex occur in milliseconds. Memories about death and the potential damage from hitting a deer register from the amygdala. Lighting-fast motor reflexes such as dropping your phone and clutching the wheel happen simultaneously. Meanwhile a cascade of biochemical events in the limbic system lead to the release of cortisol and chemical messengers that travel to the lower region of the brain and throughout the body. You begin to sweat, feel palpitations, and breathe rapidly, and if someone took a picture of your face, you'd see that your expression is as frozen as the deer in the headlights.

The activity in your prefrontal lobes just behind your forehead takes place in microseconds. The stress response takes seconds or minutes longer because of the long road it travels throughout the body.

The feeling of a near accident stays alive in you for years. Memories are the brain's storehouses of information, both learned and significant emotional events like near accidents. In order to create memories, nerve cells are thought to form new protein molecules and new interconnections. No one region of the brain stores all memories because the storage site depends on the type of memory: how to drive a car is held in motor areas, while those about smell are held in the olfactory area of the brain. The hippocampus helps the brain select where important memories will be stored. The creation of long-term memories requires attention, repetition, and associative ideas to promote new neural (synaptic) connections, such as those that are formed when practicing a sport or musical instrument. In fact, greater emotional arousal following a learning event enhances a person's retention of that event.

From an evolutionary perspective, stressful memories are stored in the brain on a subconscious level as a throwback to the ancient days when recording details of dangerous events— an encounter with a tiger or snake, for example—would lead to better ways of handling such threats in the future. Your subconscious mind (your sleeping friend or enemy) has great influence over your body. Touch someone, and many times that person will have a flashback to a past event. That's because memory is stored in the nerve cells of your body, not just your brain.

As we have seen, your brain and immune system are linked at a biochemical level, continuously signaling each other through the central nervous and immune systems. Your brain interprets the cellular production of emotions, sending this information to the "thinking" part of the brain. Cognition is our ability to process and store information about the world. We are not necessarily conscious of those activities as they occur. As we saw in the example of the near accident with the deer, many aspects of emotion rely on cognition, and cognition similarly depends on emotion.

In summary, the brain can influence the body, and the body can influence the brain. Scientists have discovered that opiate receptors are all over the body, dense in the brain, CNS, spinal cord, ANS, lungs, and abdomen. Heavy concentrations of neuropeptides live in the GI tract, skin, and muscles, including the heart. More amazingly, your own white blood cells—monocytes—manufacture neuropeptides. The monocytes speak to opiate receptors in the brain; the brain's neuropeptides speak to the body—the blood stream, heart, lungs, GI tract, urinary system, sex organs, muscles, etc. The brain is an associative network throughout the body. When you think negative thoughts, you experience negative emotions and physiological responses like the stress response. Think fear, feel fear. Emotions are biological products of the nervous system.

ACTS 2:40
And with many other words he bore witness and continued to exhort them, saying, "Save yourselves from this crooked generation."

Don't Retire to Die

HAVE YOUR RETIREMENT PARTY THE day after you die. Personally, and from the experience of others, I believe the best thing you can do to maintain mental and physical health is not to quit your job, unless you have a god-awful one. Maybe it's physically just too challenging or too stressful. If that's the case, then try to find something else to do on a daily basis, at least part-time. I say even if you're neutral to the job, keep it. It brings in some extra money, gives you reason to get out of bed, improves your self-esteem, and keeps you among the people and your friends and social contacts. If you decide to retire, if you can find a job that helps other people, that is especially invigorating and gives you a purpose in life. That's a very good thing to have as you're getting older. It increases neurogenesis, the growth of brain cells, and it increases synotogenisis, the growth of your synapses, which will improve your memory and mental functioning.

You will live longer, stay mentally alert longer, have less illness, and be a lot happier. I've heard that so often in my practice. Yesterday morning I had a cup of coffee at Starbucks. I was writing a chapter for this book, and I said hello to a gentleman I see there every day having a cup of coffee. He is retired, and I think he finds socialization at the coffee shop. I had been seeing him there for at least a year. I was talking to him about my chapter on not retiring. He said, "Doc, you're absolutely right. Last year a friend of mine had just cut his cake at a little retirement party at GM. Within one hour of that, he went to the infirmary with chest pain and was dead from a heart attack within a few hours." It's an unfortunate but true story, and I have heard that scenario before. Many die within two to four years of retirement although they are still relatively young.

When you work at something that you enjoy, it is not work. I don't consider doing neurosurgery at age seventy-four, writing books, and giving a lot of lectures to be work. It's the engine of my life. I saw two of my old friends having dinner at a restaurant the other night; one sells cars and the other runs a company. They were both in their mid-seventies. Their wives had died, and they both had dates, and they looked very healthy. What can you say—examples tell the story.

If you're not working, you probably will slow down, sit behind the TV, and start eating the sad, mad, toxic American diet. There will be a payoff. Then again, others find a job they always wanted to do, and it's very good for them. But let's face it: finding another job in your sixties is not easy. Some take the opportunity and start doing workouts. They didn't do it before on a regular basis. That's wonderful, but not a common story. You must fire it and wire it, use it or lose it.

Jack LaLanne, the famous exercise teacher, says, "Don't retire." He's working at age ninety-six. "I will push to my last breath," he says. I recommend that you read his recent book. When you retire you'll soon be looking for something to do; your ego goes down. "What am I good for today?" "Who needs me?"

Most people die within five years of retirement. A good retirement is about a two-week vacation. If your job is too risky for your age, then find another one if you can. As mentioned previously, finding a job helping other people has established my purpose in life, which is very important. I feel very blessed in that regard. The wonderful feel of a week of work, or a vacation—I'm sure you can remember that. Anticipating it will not come back if you're not working. For example, Memorial Day weekend starts tomorrow, and I'm going to the lake for three and a half days. I've been looking forward to it for a couple of weeks. It's a wonderful feeling you can only get when you're working.

After your retirement, you'll be missing work, as most people do, and may start to develop some health problems. I hope not. The potential for the development of bad habits, lack of exercise, and overeating could develop.

Jack LaLanne knows a gym owner whose retirement lasted six months. The gym owner said, "Jack, you know there were a lot of problems, but sometimes it's better to have problems than none at all. It makes you feel alive." Jack LaLanne towed seventy boats across the Queensway Bay Bridge on his seventieth birthday. While swimming in chains.

I was seventy-four April 25. I'm writing four books at the same time; playing tennis three to four days a week; practicing full-time neurosurgery, including taking emergency night calls; practicing music every week; and talking to a lot of people every day, and I'm happy to say I feel great and have no significant health problems. Incidentally, I weigh 155 pounds and follow an 80 percent vegan diet. I'm training to play in the seventy-five-and-over national tennis tournament. Tennis has been a love of mine for decades—besides my lovely wife, of course. I also have a one-hour weekly TV show, which is all about wellness. What's the point? Fire it and wire it, use it or lose it.

My wife says, "Don't retire. When would you wear all those fancy ties and suits?" All day I hear from patients while walking the hospital, "You look great, Doc." I heal people, but they heal me in return, big time. A loving doctor who looks healthy can heal a lot of people with a placebo effect. Believe me, it's worked for me for years. At least 50 percent of patients can be healed by good coaching. My patients know I love them. I'm a placebo, but they are a placebo to me. I can't imagine not being a doctor and going to work.

MATTHEW 24:22

And if those days had not been cut short, no human being would be saved. But for the sake of the elect those days will be cut short.

The Best of Dr. Rudy's Motivation Principles

THE RUDY IN YOU IS a great book about motivation to success in sports by Rudy Ruetigger. You may have seen the movie, which was about building teamwork, fair play, and sportsmanship.

But my name is Rudy too. A lot of the principles laid down by Notre Dame's Rudy are actually what I teach to motivate success and wellness. Of the forty or so most powerful motivators, I would like to pick the top ten, to my way of thinking.

Before I do that, I would like to tell you the story of my interest in motivation. Recently I was the guest speaker at a National Chiropractic Association meeting. I gave my talk on reversing type 2 diabetes by eating a proper diet, and a very nice chiropractic doctor stood up and said, "Thank you. The information is great, but how do I motivate my patients to follow it?" I think that's a very fair question, and I decided to read a lot about it and write a book about it, as this information has only limited value if people don't use it to become well.

Why does Dr. Rudy (me) have such a great interest in the teaching of wellness? For one, all my life I've had a great interest in playing sports of all types. I was not a natural athlete at anything. As a matter of fact, in high school I used to have to try to gain weight. In grade school and high school, I always tried to join a sports team—all the sports. I lived in New York City and played at Central Park every day—handball, tennis, and baseball. I tried very hard to become good at sports, but my ability was limited. Let's say at best, it was a little bit above average. My father had no interest in sports. He worked in his delicatessen day and night. Only through a lot of practice did I get good enough to make the baseball team, basketball team, and, yes, even the football team. I had a lot of help, as it was a small school. I weighed only 135 pounds, but playing sports certainly was a good step to wellness. I was not an overweight teenager. My parents consistently ate the wrong deli food—fat, sugary, and salty food. They were both overweight.

The teaching of exercise and nutrition was not part of medical school, and it barely is now. I was at my forty-fifth medical school reunion recently, and they asked if anyone had any questions. There were three female medical students at the luncheon, and I asked them how much they had learned about nutrition and wellness. All three said very little. That was a very sad day for me, and it still has not changed.

After I started my practice and looked closely at my patients' medical problems—remember, I'm a neurosurgeon—I developed a sense early in my practice that the majority of illnesses and diseases I was looking at were self-inflicted. Stress, lack of exercise, and what the patients were eating was a cause of 50 to 80 percent of what I was treating. Many were type 2 diabetics from being overweight. That could be simply corrected by being the proper weight. Then I found a book, *How to Live 365 Days a Year*, by Dr. Schindler. I handed out about five thousand copies free to my patients. My corporation took about $3000 off my quarterly bonuses to pay for it. And I was happy to do it. A lot of patients get well without injections, medications, or surgery. I felt

I was a doctor doing what was right. After all, the word physician means teacher. We are not graduating teachers from the medical school.

Eventually I read everything I could get my hands on about wellness and found out that, frankly, it's all interrelated, and my knowledge base grew tremendously. My motivation to teach this on a wider scale flew off the charts. I don't seem to be able to keep quiet about it, no matter where I go. I now have a wellness center with a yoga studio. We teach proper eating, exercise, individual and group training, meditation, stress reduction, dancing, and many other programs. My website is ***www. KachmannMindBody.com***. By December I will probably have ten published books in every aspect of wellness. I developed the Mind-Body Index, a list of illnesses caused partially or totally by the mind, usually stress. I made about twenty CDs and DVDs, one-hour lectures on the effects of the mind on the human body, about stress, cancer, exercise, proper eating, the nocebo effect, etc. I give at least thirty lectures a year on wellness and have a one-hour weekly TV show about wellness that attracts a large audience.

Clearly, it was a love of teaching the patient how to get well without having to give him dangerous medications or doing surgery that inspired me. Really, it's about love for the patients, the ability to make them well in the safest manner and reducing the amount of illness and disease that they have and increasing their longevity.

My Top Ten Motivators

1. Food—what we eat
2. Life-changing events
3. Visualization and imaging
4. Commitment
5. Power of positive thinking
6. Mind-body connection
7. The will to live
8. Meditation
9. Yoga and chi-gung
10. Purpose

We all have different things that motivate us. Take a moment to write down ten things that motivate you the most below.

1 _____

2_____

3 _____

4 _____

5 _____

6 _____

7 _____

8_____

9 _____

10_____

MATTHEW 24:13

But the one who endures to the end will be saved.

Avoid Risky Behavior

Courage is almost a contradiction in terms. It means a strong desire to live, taking the form of readiness to die.

–G. K. CHESTERTON

Courage is resistance to fear, mastery of fear—not absence of fear. Except a creature is part coward it is not a compliment to say it is brave.

–Mark Twain

THE QUOTES ABOVE MAY SEEM like unusual maxims to begin the Third Prescription, but hopefully it will become clear why I have selected statements about courage when avoiding undue risks. I was privileged to serve my country as an officer in the US Navy during the Vietnam War. As a neurosurgeon I witnessed and attended to many young soldiers with serious injuries. Today we are witnessing soldiers returning from Iraq with injuries that they will carry for the rest of their lives, wounds that were the result of the risk they took to bring forth liberty for the citizens of Iraq. I want to commend the brave soldiers of our coalition for the risks they have taken and the courage they have exhibited. Their sacrifices were surely coupled with intense fears they had to face and conquer in order to pursue a greater good.

This is the challenge: convincing youth that they are not invincible and that they must treat life with care by avoiding undue risks. First you must understand that I deal daily with people who have been rushed to the emergency room. Their brains, and the potential to think and create and imagine, may never again function with proficiency because a helmet was overlooked and a risk was taken. Legs will never again be used for running, dancing, or even to walk; arms that could have hugged and held, or fingers that would have written poems, drawn sketches, painted pictures, and played musical instruments will never again function because a seat belt was not worn; or a reckless dive into shallow water snaps a neck, and now I stand with a family who will have to care for their loved one for the rest of their lives.

While I was writing this book, a very unfortunate accident took place. A young man in the prime of his life, named Noel, was standing on the bed of a pickup truck. It was certainly a risky choice, and that careless moment resulted in a lifetime of grave adversity. Young Noel was flipped from the truck and landed headfirst on the ground, resulting in a tragic brain injury. I am pleased to say that Noel is making great progress in his rehabilitation and will be able to participate in the Wheel Chair Athletic Foundation that I have established in the Tri-State area for just such unfortunate men and women. I am reminded, each time I see Noel in an office visit, of the importance of treating life with care and avoiding risky behavior.

For as long as I can remember in my medical practice, deaths have occurred because:

Drugs and alcohol were abused.

Seatbelts were not fastened (more than one half of the young drivers killed in car accidents were not wearing seatbelts).

Motorcycles were recklessly ridden.

Guns were not protected from children or were used violently in an argument.

Wave runners were used without careful instructions being followed.

Every day of my practice, I have to stand with grieving families who have lost a father, mother, son, or daughter. If they aren't grief stricken over a loss by death, they are facing the permanent disability of a once-active member of their home.

An October 19, 2003 *Parade* magazine article gave a staggering statistic:

Firearms kill eight children or teenagers each day. An American child is twelve times more likely to die from gunfire than a child in any other industrialized nation.

Certainly we should not be thwarted from approaching our vast reservoirs of potential because the roads are guarded by dragons of fear. Fear has barred far too many from enjoying life, causing them to miss experiences that could enhance the quality of their lives. Most definitely we stand in appreciation for risks taken with courage, in the midst of fear, by our sons and daughters in times of war. I acknowledge that each time I sit behind the wheel of a car, I am taking a risk and that I must conquer fear or I would never leave home. But I treat life with care by fastening my seatbelt, obeying traffic laws, shutting off the cell phone, and driving as defensively as possible.

As Mark Twain said, "We need to have courage to face, resist, and master our fears." I do not believe that this is best illustrated by MTV's program *Jackass*, which challenges people to perform stunts that could maim them for life. The network reality show *Fear Factor* is not instilling courage in our lives either, but rather is distorting our value of our most treasured possession—the gift of life. This gift is far too precious to risk it with dangerous choices. It is my sincere belief that the mind is clouded and good choices obscured when it is affected by the destructive influence of alcohol and drugs. I will discuss this further later in the book, but this prescription could not be fairly presented without exposing the reality of the dangers that substance abuse has on the careless disregard for life in making choices that involve risky behavior.

ISAIAH 40:22
It is he who sits above the circle of the earth, and its inhabitants are like grass-hoppers; who stretches out the heavens like a curtain, and spreads them like a tent to dwell in;

Positive Thinking

WHEN YOU HAVE WHAT IT takes to deal creatively and not destructively with the sometimes harsh fact of human existence and still believe in good outcomes, you are a tough-minded, optimistic, real positive thinker. To have resiliency under the application of force and not break apart, to have a good, substantial texture of personality, that is to be tough in the face of danger. When you are tough, you can endure strain and not break apart in your thoughts. A psychiatrist said, "The chief duty of man is to endure life." But he told only half the story, and the poorer half at that. To be tough-minded, we are actually optimists. When we are tough-minded optimists and positive thinkers, then we are people who do not break apart with negative thoughts; we continue to be hopeful and cheerful and expect the good, no matter what the apparent situation is.

Let's face it: to live in this world, you have just got to be strong. Without strength, you will get crushed or at least crumble. Some would even say life eventually is a catastrophe for everyone. But let's enjoy the ride. Think of all the things that can happen to people in general—pain, sickness, frustration, death, accidents, diseases, illnesses, job loss, failure, divorce, and double-dealing.

Something will get you sometime; that lets you develop real inner resistance, and it will rock you. Tough mindedness is a quality of top priority. We have the instinct to be tough minded within all of us. It is put in our bodies in evolution. There is a doctor living within all of us. We just need to know how to tap into him. That's what I am trying to teach you.

Frank Leahy, one-time football coach at Notre Dame, wrote on the locker room wall, "When the going gets tough, the tough get going." See yourself not as a weak, wishy-washy, and vacillating person but as a strong, controlled, purposeful individual. You tend to become just what you picture yourself to be. To help visualize yourself in terms of the strong mental pattern, I suggest daily use of the following affirmation. An affirmation is a positive statement reinforcing what you are thinking. "God made me strong. I see myself as I really am—strong. Thank you, God, for my strength."

Keep saying this, keep thinking this, and keep believing this. In due course your conscious mind will accept your affirmations as fact. You are what your subconscious mind really believes you are. You have within you all the strength you need to handle anything you will ever have to face. Every human being becomes what he pictures himself as being. Don't ever let your mind control you. You always can control it.

WHAT IT TAKES TO TAKE TO BE TOUGH

1. *The strong develop inner toughness.*
2. *When things get tough, the tough get going.*
3. *Constantly reemphasize to yourself the great fact that God built potential strength into your nature.*
4. *Get in touch with your spirituality.*
5. *Reverse your mental image of yourself as being weak to a clear picture of yourself as becoming stronger.*
6. *Practice until you master it.*
7. *Become a positive thinker.*

8. *Know for a fact that with God's help, you can take what you have to take courageously and victoriously.*
9. *Remember, what you think you will become.*
10. *"Haven't I commanded you? Strength! Courage! Don't be timid; don't get discouraged. GOD, your God, is with you every step you take." (Josh. 1:9)*

WORK ON THE MASTERY OF FEAR

Always wrap medicine and religion together into a kind of body, mind, and soul package. Dr. Norman Vincent Peale, the famous minister and authors father did just that. I have read over twenty-one books written by Dr. Norman Vincent Peale, essentially all about positive thinking. I recommend his books highly. He clearly connects spirituality and healing. As the mind is healed, so are the body and soul, according to Dr. Peale. He states after studying people who overcame cancer, alcoholism, diseases, illnesses, psychological problems, "It was in almost any case an in-depth surrender to their God." When you think of it, that is very similar to the twelve principles of Alcoholics Anonymous. Dr. Peale found that a basic fact in living without fear is to practice the simple belief in your God, and he will take care of you, in that you do everything within your power to also help yourself. Ninety percent of fear is never realized. Get rid of your fears. Certainly the first reaction to the diagnosis of cancer many times is unbearable fear—fully understandable. What you have to do, which I would say is the first essential step, is surrender, or let go and let God take control . Remember that's one of the first steps that Alcoholics Anonymous also uses. You have taken steps in the presence of God; you're not alone. That is a doctor living within you. You must invite God's presence to lead in the healing and become positive minded. Man is what he thinks, not what he says, reads, or hears. You can free yourself from any chain, whether poverty, pain, ill health, unhappiness, or fear.

FAITH IS STRONGER THAN FEAR

1. *Never be afraid of anything or anybody.*
2. *Have a sound, rugged set of beliefs.*
3. *Change your life from fear to faith, and fear will pass away.*

"Your soul is dyed the color of your thoughts," Tolstoy said. "To know God is to live." Look for the white cloud and drop the dark view. Become a tough-minded optimist. Muster up your character. The magic of enthusiasm can work magic in your life. Whatever happens, whatever losses you have, your combat capacity will keep working, and all of us have this comeback potential. There is a deep tendency in human nature to become precisely what we imagine ourselves as being. Hold certain images in your consciousness like a photograph. The human capacity to use visualization imaging for memory and positive neurochemistry is unlimited. We become what we picture. Storms always pass by, and the glory of God shines through. Always make yourself enthusiastic; get in the habit of thinking happy thoughts.

Faith says the doctors function is to get you into a better frame of mind, and you can mobilize your hormones, neurotransmitters, neuropeptides and your army, navy, and air force to heal you. Resentment can have ill effects. Everything you resent only accentuates the hurt and interferes with healing. Free yourself from unhealthy thoughts.

POSITIVE THOUGHTS AND HEALING

It must be a real desire, real faith, and a sincere reaching out with all your mind, body, and spirit to promote the healing power. This comprehensive breakout of self will break through the barrier of resentment, hatred, anxiety, and depression, which will flow the great force of healing and good health.

PRAYER, LOVE, FAITH AND POSITIVE THINKING CAN LEAD TO HEALING

1. *Establish a spiritual team of like-minded friends.*
2. *Use the power of a spiritual commitment.*
3. *Take spiritual authority over the malignant cells. Use a healer to help you.*
4. *Remember Luke 9:1: "When Jesus had called the Twelve together, he gave them power and authority to drive out all demons and to cure diseases"—Healthy thoughts (or use your own religious healing).*
5. *Use highly recommended oncology treatments.*
6. *Find a great physician.*

Every morning say, "Isn't this a glorious bad morning?" Even if it's icy, snowing, or stormy. Religion is a path to spirituality and accepting things as they are. Optimism is positive thinking with a light bulb on. The positive figure is a hardheaded, tough-minded, and factual realist. He sees all the difficulties, and I mean all. What can be said for the average negative thinker? The positive thinker, unlike the negative, does not allow difficulties and problems to depress him—and certainly not to defeat him. He looks expectantly beyond all and acknowledges difficulties for creative solutions. In other words, he sees more than difficulties; he tries to see the solutions of those difficulties.

The positive thinker is completely objective. He has definite goals. He never takes no for an answer, almost always pulling through. And even if he doesn't, he has the satisfaction of knowing he gave it a good try, which is something, a mighty satisfying something. Be glad you have problems—they are a sign of life. If you have no problems, I doubt you're living

The Spiritual Connection

REMEMBER, SPIRITUAL HEALING IS PART of mind-body healing. Spiritual imaging encourages us to experience a direct connection with the divine, in whatever way we except divinity. This imaging can project a prospective wider view of the mystic, encouraging miracles to happen.

SPIRITUAL GUIDED IMAGERY

Spiritual imagery is imaging that encourages us to experience a direct connection with the divine, in whatever way we experience divinity. This can be in the service of helping us with our view of ourselves, our connection to our own life for life's purpose of renewing our perception of ourselves as part of everyone and everything. In other words, this is imaging that can offer us perspective from the wider point of view of the mystic.

To begin with, make yourself comfortable. Position yourself so that your head, neck, and spine are straight, shifting your weight so that your body feels supported. Take in a couple full, deep, cleansing breaths, inhaling as fully as you comfortably can, sending the warm energy of your breath to any part of your body that is sore or tense or tight and releasing the discomfort so that you can feel your breath going to all those tight, tense places, and then gathering up all the tension and breathing it out so that more and more you can feel safe and comfortable, relaxed and easy, watching and feeling your heart open to a warmth that expands into your entire chest softly and easily and alter your body, touching an ancient memory of who you really are and who you always have been and always will be, touching your own bright, indestructible soul. Held by deep understanding and a sense of utter safety, you can take in fully and deeply the loves that are freely offered to you as you feel your own love in return, free and boundless. Understanding that in this powerful circuitry between you, it's the same love that fills you both, that the giver is a receiver and the receiver is the source. See the beauty of your life and comprehend your own life journey from the vantage of this powerful, healing light, seeing it all. All the pain and fear, the courage, kindness, love, the special gifts of abilities, the moments of triumph and great beauty, the moments of despair and loss of perspective—all of it seen through the softness of this exquisite light. Feel a new kindness toward yourself and others, the new forgiveness of yourself and others for disappointments of the past, letting it go and making room for possibility and growth.

Mindfulness, Meditation and Healing

MINDFULNESS IS A STATE OF mind in which the mind is solely focused on what is happening, focusing on one thing and not allowing itself to wander.

When this is done, a deep calm pervades both body and mind, a state of mind that needs to be experienced to be understood. Meditation is a way of doing it. Mindfulness can be applied to everything that we do—speeding, driving, doing the dishes, working, and playing. There are endless ways to meditate.

The meditator focuses on a certain item, chant, light, word, or object. It results in relaxation and even a state of rapture. Pain may go away, and pathological thinking may change. Visualizing a change may eliminate a bad habit. Mindfulness is stripping the baggage off the main thing we're dealing with in that moment. No past, no future, no worry or anxiety. True reductionist reasoning, the bare facts. You're concentrating to strip off the wall of the illusions that block living in reality. It strips the baggage accompanying pain, or bad habits, the baggage that causes us to smoke, be fearful, and develop toxic habits.

Mindfulness can be liberating—just the bare facts. The breath is generally used as a method of connecting the mind and the body and is the object of our concentration. Life is a catastrophe, let's face it. In the end it's always a tragedy. Life is incessant with constant change; nothing lasts forever. So to constantly act as if we're living in a continuous catastrophe is a mistake. We need to learn to live in the moment. Practicing mindfulness and meditation is very helpful. It's the nature of the universe that nothing stays the same. We're too judgmental. Stop judging everything; it's stressful. Everything is not just good, bad, or neutral. Things blend into one another, according to the Tao, the Chinese way of thinking. The essence of life is suffering, say the Buddhists. Happiness and peace are really the prime issues in human existence. This is what we are seeking, but we cover up with issues, and you can learn to step outside of this cycle of wants and desires.

Meditation is intended to purify the mind. It can change the thought process of what we call psychic irritations—greed, hatred, jealousy. Meditation brings the mind to a state of tranquility, awareness, concentration, and insight. Meditation is a great teacher. It's like cultivating a new land. Mindful meditation brings together certain attitudes that are essential. We are heading for the bottom line; the truth for the moment. Don't expect anything. Meditational mindful awareness seeks to see reality exactly as it is. Feel through pain, without its baggage, a suspension of all preconceived ideas. No judgment. Let go, accept anything that arises—no hopelessness or obsession, and above all, no judgment. Question everything except reality. View all problems as challenges. Don't dwell or obsess about anything.

Start mindful meditation by focusing on your breath. Pay attention to every aspect of breathing in practicing mindfulness. You want to practice mindfulness and calm the mind by developing insight and wisdom to realign the truth as it is. You want to know the work of the mind as it really is. You want to get rid of all psychic irritations and annoyances and make your life truly peaceful and happy. Your mind cannot be purified without seeing things as they really are. We should not confuse them with mental formations for body sensations in complexities of the mind. We need to separate the mind and body feelings. When we mindfully watch both body and mind, we can see how many wonderful things they do together.

Mindful practice is the practice of being 100 percent truthful with ourselves. If we are mindful, we will be diligent, so we need to look into our own mind.

We will be thankful if someone points out our faults. Before we try to surmount our defects, we should know what they are.

Even when we are suffering, we can pretend we are not, or we will not get better. If we are blind to all faults, someone needs to point them out to us. If one becomes unmindful of one's faults, that person will not become better. We should speak mindfully and live mindfully. When we are listening and talking mindfulness, our minds are free from greed, selfishness, hatred, and delusion.

Mindfulness is the English translation of the Pali word *sati*. It is an activity. It was introduced by the Buddha twenty-five centuries ago and is a set of mental activities, specifically a sphere and the state of uninterrupted mindfulness. We have developed the habit of squandering and decorating our thoughts with baggage, causing a great deal of stress. Label it, and most of all, get involved in a long string of symbolic thought about it. Using proper techniques prolongs mindfulness; you find this experience is profound in that it changes your entire view of the universe. The state of this section is to be learned; however, it takes regular practice.

Mindfulness is mirror thought. It reflects only what is presently happening in exactly the way it is happening. There are no biases. Mindfulness is nonjudgmental observation. It is the ability of the mind to observe without criticism. With this ability, one sees things without condemnation or judgment. One does not decide and does not judge. Mindfulness is an impartial watchfulness. It takes no sides. Mindfulness does not get infatuated with good mental states, and it does not try to sidestep bad mental states. You can use it to break every sort of bad habit you may have. Mindless thieves all expenses equally, all thoughts equally, all feelings equally. Nothing is suppressed. Mindfulness does not play favorites. Mindfulness is not conceptual awareness. It is bare attention, it is not thinking. It does not get involved with thoughts of concepts. It does not get hung up on ideas or opinions of memories. Mindfulness registers experiences but does not compare them. Mindfulness is present-moment awareness. Mindfulness is non-egotistic awareness. One just sits back and watches the show. Mindfulness is the observance of the basic nature of each passing phenomenon. Mindfulness works like an electron microscope. Mindfulness actually sees the character of every perception. It sees the transitory and passing nature of everything that is observed.

Apply your attention to the proper object at the proper time and exert precisely the amount of energy needed to do that job. When this energy is properly applied, meditative states reveal a state of calm alertness. There's no greed, lust, or laziness. Be prepared. In the mind there lies a mechanism that accepts what the mind expands. This is beautiful and pleasant, and it rejects experiences that are perceived as ugly and painful. This mechanism gives rise to the states of mind that we are training ourselves to avoid.

Mindfulness is attention to present-moment reality and is therefore directly the opposite of the day's state of mind that characterizes impediments. Fully developed mindfulness is a state of total nonattachment and utter absence of clinging to anything in the world. It sees things deeply, down below the level of concepts and opinions. The result is a mind that remains unstained and invulnerable, completely undisturbed by the ups and downs of life. The point is that we can use mindfulness to bring happiness, stop toxic habits, develop good health habits, and have a happy, long life with a sound mind.

Sleep for Good Brain Function

MOST AMERICANS ARE IN DEBT—NOT from bills, but from lack of sleep. Sleep debt percolates over time and must be repaid, or it will accumulate and interfere with the proper function of your brain.

You have difficulty getting up in the morning, fall asleep at the breakfast table, are irritable to the family, make poor decisions, lack energy, are grouchy and unpleasant to be around, and even fall asleep at the wheel while driving to work—not a good start on your day. A lot of America operates that way. We're just too busy. Your memory acts as if it's impaired. No brain works well on sleep debt. People without proper sleep become more forgetful, paranoid, anxious, and depressed. They make poor decisions.

Our hippocampus and the temporal lobe convert short-term memory to long-term memory when we are asleep. So sleep is very necessary and important for good long-term memory.

Our brain is actually working while we are asleep. There are many stages of sleep. Our brain waves have many different forms when we are asleep. This was extensively studied by Dr. William C. Dement, who published a very good book called *The Promise of Sleep*.

Sleep apnea, a stoppage in breathing during sleep, can be very dangerous. It is more common in overweight people. People with this problem are more likely to develop high blood pressure, heart disease, and strokes. They also have memory problems and are more likely to develop dementia. Although I'm a neurosurgeon, I see people with this frequently, and they need to be referred to a sleep center for study. We need one hour of sleep for every two hours of wakefulness. When the brain is asleep, it is not resting at all. It's busy at work while the rest of our body may be resting.

Dreaming permits each and every one of us to be quietly and safely insane every night of our lives, says Dr. Dement. Dr. Dement says, "Sleeping brains are like soldiers in the battlefield." And now they're locked in a vicious biological combat between the powerful and opposing drives of the brain cells and the biochemistry of the body with different agendas. Sleep is just not located in the head, but actually involves every corner of the body.

We have an internal clock, the suprachiasmatic nucleus, which regulates our sleep habits, the circadian rhythm. It works even if you're living in a cave, for it is also called process C. It stimulates the hormones and chemicals that put us asleep. Larks wake up early and go to bed early. As an example, night owls who go to bed late and get up early have huge sleep debt. Sleep has been shown to enhance tasks that involve visual texture, discrimination, motor adaptation, and motor sequencing. Learning a new procedure is most sensitive to sleep. Learning new tasks decreases in quality when you are in sleep debt. The bottom line is sleep debt means brain function flaws. Sleep loss cripples thinking. People with sleep debt don't live as long, and they don't learn as well and have poor memory. Sleep debt results in loss of immediate memory, decreased mood, loss of logical reasoning ability, and decreased sexual function. Eventually sleep also affects manual dexterity. Sleep is intimately involved with learning and memory. To live a long life and have a good functioning brain requires adequate sleep.

LUKE 21:36

But stay awake at all times, praying that you may have strength to escape all these things that are going to take place, and to stand before the Son of Man."

MORE FROM DR. KACHMANN

Books:

Pain – We Need a New Definition
The Fraud of Chronic Pain
Healing Cancer With The Power Of Your Mind
Live To Be 100 With a Sound Mind and Body
The Call of Life
The Fraud of Alzheimer's Disease (also available on DVD)
Nocebo: Placebo's Evil Twin (also available on DVD and CD)
The Secret of the Non Diet for Adults (also available on DVD and CD)
The Secret of the Non Diet for Children (also available on DVD and CD)
Kid Scripts: Just What the Doctor Ordered
The Psychology of Eating (also available on DVD and CD)
Reversing Type 2 Diabetes in 60 Days (also available on DVD and CD)
Welcome to Your Mind Body (also available on DVD and CD)
Secrets of Motivating Yourself to Wellness (also available on DVD and CD)

And more, visit www.amazon.com

DVDs:
The Mind and Stress (also available on CD)
Living Healthier and Longer (also available on CD)
Chinese Medicine (also available on CD)
Acute and Chronic Pain (also available on CD)
Smoking Cessation (also available on CD)
True Vitality (DVD only)

Secrets of the Mind and Cancer (DVD only)

And more, visit www.amazon.com

www.ingramcontent.com/pod-product-compliance
Lightning Source LLC
Chambersburg PA
CBHW070009300526
45794CB00001B/248